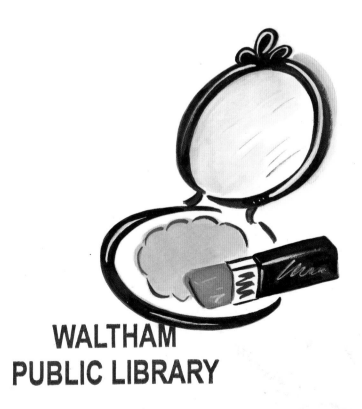

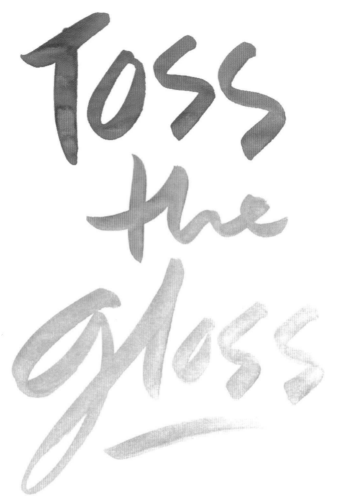

Toss the gloss

Beauty Tips, Tricks & Truths for Women 50+

ANDREA Q. ROBINSON

Illustrated by Chesley McLaren

SEAL PRESS

Page 4 photo credits: top right © Alex Chatelain, *Vogue France*, October 1969; bottom right © Eric Boman,
Vogue Australia, November 1993; bottom left © Jennifer Livingston, *Women's Wear Daily*, 2002.

ISBN 978-1-58005-621-2

Library of Congress Cataloging-in-Publication Data

Robinson, Andrea Q.,
Toss the gloss : beauty tips, tricks, and truths for women 50+.
pages cm
ISBN 978-1-58005-621-2
1. Women–Health and hygiene. 2. Middle-aged women–Health and hygiene.
3. Beauty, Personal. I. Title. II. Title: Beauty tips, tricks, and truths
for women 50+.
RA778.R5288 2014
646.7'2–dc23
2013040180

Published by
Seal Press
An imprint of Perseus Books
A division of Hachette Book Group
1700 Fourth Street
Berkeley, California
sealpress.com

9 8 7 6 5 4 3 2 1

Cover design by Erin Seaward-Hiatt and Domini Dragoone
Interior design by meganjonesdesign.com
Printed in China by RR Donnelley
Distributed by Publishers Group West

With love for my mother, the dreamer; my daughter, the naturalist; and my son, the realist. Dazzling inspirations, all of them.

CONTENTS

What's that you say, MRS. Robinson?

INTRODUCTION

HOW MUCH TIME DO YOU HAVE, DEAR READER, BECAUSE I HAVE GOT A LOT TO SAY. WHY LISTEN? BECAUSE I'VE SPENT DECADES RUNNING BEAUTY COMPANIES:

Ultima II, Ralph Lauren, Tom Ford, and Prescriptives, to name just a few. And I'm here to blow the whistle on the beauty industry and give you the real scoop on the business—the good, the bad, and the ugly.

I've tried it all. I've seen it all. I know too much.

Think of me as your personal cosmetics guinea pig. In the name of beauty (and many, many jobs in the beauty industry), I've tried everything out there: lotions, makeup, injections, spas, lasers, you name it. Once I even tried crushed beetle skin on my face, just to test the truth of the Indian legend that extols its youth-preserving magical properties. (As it turned out, it didn't work, but I think you'll agree, that was real commitment!)

After years in the beauty trenches, I've acquired the ultimate beauty industry insider's perspective, and I'm ready to spill it all—even if it means inciting a powder-puff fatwa.

How do I know all these whispered truths? Let's just say it started where all good secrets do: at *Vogue* magazine. Back in the days before The Devil Wore Prada, I was The Beauty Editor Who Wore Revlon . . . and CoverGirl and Lancôme and Maybelline and all the rest. It was my job to try everything, from lipsticks to liposuction, and then report on it. Yes, I tried it all in the name of beauty, and no, you can't see my before and after shots. But thanks to my editor, Grace Mirabella, who reclaimed *Vogue* from a fantasy fashion magazine and made it a bible for real working women who had families and day jobs, I was able to extend her modern point of view on to *Vogue*'s beauty pages and address the needs of real women and their beauty issues.

From my perch at the magazine, I was immersed in the very best the cosmetics industry had to offer, and I spent years testing, comparing, and judging. Then, an unconventional beauty industry executive offered me a job outside *Vogue*'s chic gray walls, and I became president of Ultima II. My job was to reinvent the brand on every level—from product, to packaging, to its image in department stores and in advertising.

> How does a girl from an all-women Catholic college, where I practiced pouring tea and holding polite conversation, learn to do battle in the corporate world? I'll tell you how.

The only problem? The male executives in my office. If you think they're a pain in the butt in the boardroom, imagine a group of chauvinistic guys in suits telling you—the only female president in the corporation—that the makeup you've invented won't appeal to women just like you. This was my first business venture (or should I say, adventure), where men, whose only "cosmetic" was deodorant, were telling me what I wanted in my makeup bag! Well, let's just say they didn't know who they were dealing with. A clash of wit and wills ensued: My instincts took hold and I was determined to deliver to them the non–sugar-coated truth— what we women really want, not what they think we really want. And I did.

How does a girl from an all-women Catholic college, where I practiced pouring tea and holding polite conversation, learn to do battle in the corporate world? I'll tell you how. A friend entered me in *Glamour* magazine's "10 Best Dressed College Girls" contest. I won and that's where my adventure into the "glamorous jungle" began. After graduation, I joined a pool of young college graduates at Condé Nast (the corporation that owns *Vogue*, *Glamour*, and *Vanity Fair*, among many other magazines), assisting editors with whatever they needed. We answered telephones, picked up coffee, ferried clothes to the garment district, scheduled appointments, booked lunch dates at glamorous restaurants, escorted models to the photographer's studio for fashion and beauty shoots, and even typed their children's homework—whatever they needed.

From there, I landed a permanent job working for *Mademoiselle*, where I witnessed the most remarkable explosion of creativity marching through our office each day in the form of artists like Andy Warhol, photographers such as David Bailey, writers like Joyce Carol Oates and Truman Capote, not to mention celebrities, fashion designers, rock stars—The Beatles, Janis Joplin, Grace Slick, Cher (with Sonny), to name a few—and all the top models including Twiggy. Once, I even saw Timothy Leary smoke pot with a very cool editor at the desk next to mine. Edie Locke was the editor-in-chief during that time and turned *Mademoiselle* into the "it" magazine of its time. Nonnie Moore, the legendary editor at *Mademoiselle* magazine and the quintessential modern woman, was my boss and a fabulous mentor who, during the ten years I was there before moving to *Vogue,* not only taught me the basics of editing, but also showed me, by example, how to combine career and family, and in the process also encouraged me to value my own opinions, take chances, break rules when they didn't apply, and tap into my creative talents. That's when I first began to notice the ways in which the cosmetics industry seemed singularly geared to a lack of vision when it came to the basics of addressing the needs and desires of "real women," especially "real women" with real and special needs.

Just in case I'm being too subtle, let me be clear: I believe most men running the major beauty corporations where you undoubtedly have spent a lot of money (even if you're not a cosmetics junkie like me) think you've lost it at fifty. Sure, there are exceptions—men like Ralph Lauren (I was president of his fragrance brand) and Tom Ford (I was president of his beauty company). I'd be a fool to say those men don't understand, explore, and create what real women crave for their vanity table.

> Just in case I'm being too subtle, let me be clear: Most men running the major beauty corporations where you undoubtedly have spent a lot of money think you've lost it at fifty.

But Mr. Lauren and Mr. Ford are geniuses. The fact is that most men in charge of your makeup aren't going to change your world, or even your look. You've "aged out" of their makeup market. The only products they're spending big bucks to market to you are wrinkle creams. Sorry, ladies, but it's true.

But you can't—we can't—listen to them. You, your life, your brain, and—yes, dammit—your looks are at their prime. I know

Pictures from the fashion, beauty, and corporate worlds taken throughout my career, showing the evolution of my style: natural looking makeup and hair.

Clockwise: Vogue France, Vogue Australia, Women's Wear Daily.

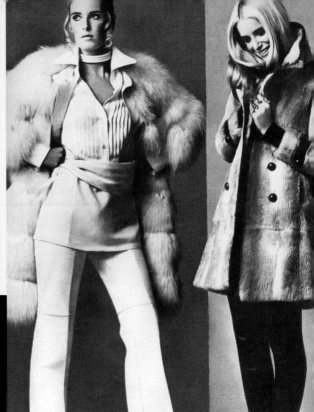

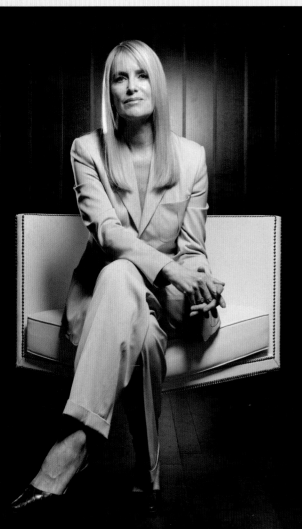

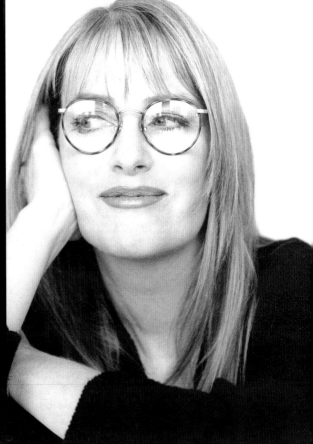

you're just as concerned as ever with looking your best. Want a pair of Manolo Blahnik shoes? How about that sexy little black dress? Who doesn't? So why wouldn't you put your money toward grown-up cosmetics to match?

The depressing, oh-go-to-hell answer for why we don't even have the opportunity to buy cosmetics geared to the color and texture of our menopausal skin is quite simple. Even if there's money to be made, the people running these corporations are afraid to address our specific needs with anything other than antiaging creams because they are worried that they will alienate their younger consumer base, even though we—the fifty+ "real women"—are the largest demographic, with more money to spend. They need to wake up and realize that we're worth their investment.

The disconnect between the industry and us really dawned on me when I accepted a job at Revlon—my first position on the corporate side of the beauty industry. There I relaunched Ultima II with the help of my *Vogue* collaborator, revered photographer Irving Penn. We created a print ad that heralded the start of something new. We set up the shoot so that each letter that spelled out U-L-T-I-M-A got its own makeup item, a visual feast of smeared lipstick, crushed eye shadow, streaked nail polish, and scribbled lip liner. Until then, beauty ads featured either provocative "babes" in overdone makeup or uptight matrons wearing ruffled blouses. The corporate execs didn't get it—frankly, they were shocked, and the ad almost didn't run. But it did, thanks to my persuasive skills with my immediate boss and the company chairman and owner, Ronald Perelman, who overruled the decision that the suits who were running his company made. And soon cash registers were ringing up sales faster than Viagra in a retirement community.

That was just the beginning. Remember "The Nakeds"? It was a groundbreaking line of thirty-eight neutral shades of makeup that predates any of the cosmetic companies that followed, including Bobbi Brown. I created that concept at Revlon. I collaborated on this project with Kevyn Aucoin, the shy, lumbering, young makeup artist from Louisiana who helped me with shade selection and would become the biggest makeup artist name in the industry. And I created it because my mission in the beauty business was to help women *look like themselves, only better.* I had to fight the corporate machine to even get the collection on the counters, but, when it arrived in the stores, women loved it, and it sold out everywhere. "Why would a woman want to wear mud on

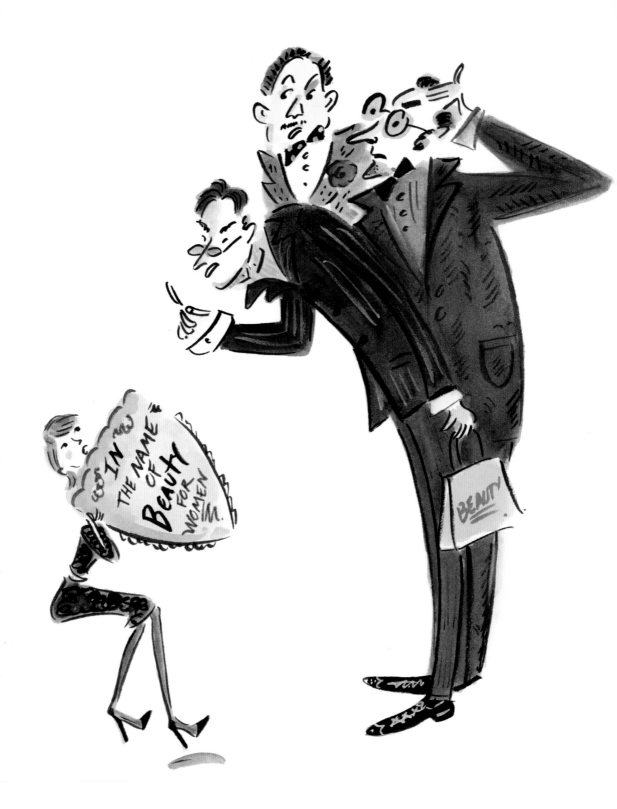

her face?" the suits asked. "Makeup is about disguise and fantasy." This was 1990, and women had been flooding the workplace with their blue eye shadow, pink lipstick, and orange cheeks—can you imagine? It was war paint for girls (created by men)—for an entire decade. The Nakeds became a cultural statement as well as a fashion statement. Women wholeheartedly embraced the idea of looking like themselves, only better. The concept made millions and catapulted me to the next phase of my career. More important, it catapulted the women of our generation to a new kind of sex appeal, one that relied on who we were instead of a man's fantasy.

The Nakeds were followed by the The Naughty Nakeds, and the first ever long-wearing lipstick (women could go to work and not have to think about reapplying their lipstick all day—remember, it was the '80s. Everyone wore lipstick). After that, I was lured to L'Oreal, where I had the privilege of working with Ralph Lauren and his burgeoning collection of women's fragrances. I helped Ralph create his blockbuster fragrance successes: Romance, Romance Men, Polo Blue, Polo Black, and Ralph. We also worked together on a makeup collection. While I was there, Ralph Lauren Fragrances became the largest fragrance franchise in the world.

I loved those years, but when Estée Lauder came calling again (after a thirty-year courtship on their part to hire me), I signed on. Because the company was founded by a woman, I thought it would further my mis-

> The Nakeds became a cultural statement as well as a fashion statement.

sion to work on a brand that had a built-in audience of fifty+ women who had come of age with the brand. I was named global chief marketing officer for the Estée Lauder brand, and, when Tom Ford created his own brand in the Lauder Corporation, I became its president. My responsibility as president was to help him realize his makeup and fragrance vision. Together, we launched a very successful and unique group of Private Blend fragrances for men and for women, and worked on a makeup collection that would follow later. Ironically, they fired me when I was fifty+. The suit who was running Estée Lauder said he thought it was time for me to retire. *Retire?!* I was just getting started.

WHILE MY LIFE and my career were happening, my own beauty needs were changing. Being married, raising two children, maintaining a full-time career, and supporting a household began to take its toll on my looks, which I had always taken for granted. I noticed the inevitable lines, wrinkles, and shadows under my eyes, and my once fresh-looking skin seemed to have checked out of my face and run for the hills. A visit with my mother crystallized the situation when she gently suggested that I make some time to spend on myself, inferring that I had started to look like I was "letting myself go." She said that I came last on the list when it came to my family. I laughed (probably should have cried) and remarked that I wasn't even on the list! Sound familiar? This was a seminal moment—my mother, who always thought I was beautiful (don't all mothers feel that way?), and this direct conversation prompted me to take immediate action. I was overweight, so I got a membership at the local gym (dropped twenty pounds in four months), and my family went on a healthy diet with me. I went to my dermatologist and started addressing the burgeoning needs of my skin with the Fraxel laser and fillers (more about this later), and I started playing with makeup and treatments to find a regime that would restore that lost youthfulness to my tired little face.

And somewhere between the drama of surgical scaffolding and the myth of miracle skin treatments, I discovered a potent realm of targeted, useful makeup that really works for women over fifty. And thanks to my collaboration with the cosmetic scientists, makeup artists, photographers, actresses, hairdressers, models, dermatologists, cosmetologists, plastic surgeons, witch doctors, rich doctors, and beauty junkies, I knew when and how to apply it. I began to tinker with existing products, mixing and matching formulas, and in the process created new ones geared to my needs.

If your real goal is looking like yourself, only better, this is your go-to book. The surprisingly simple truth I want to share with you, through every chapter, is this: The right makeup, used the right way, is the most powerful weapon in your beauty arsenal. Let this be your first beauty commandment. This book will serve as your guide to recapture the glamorous you. Forget about makeup reclaiming youth. Good makeup reclaims *you.* It's the Chanel in your sample sale, the Splenda in your latte, the fully charged battery in your iPad—it's the sizzle that leads to feeling good and confident; it's instant gratification and major fun, and I'm going to help you get it. Let's go!

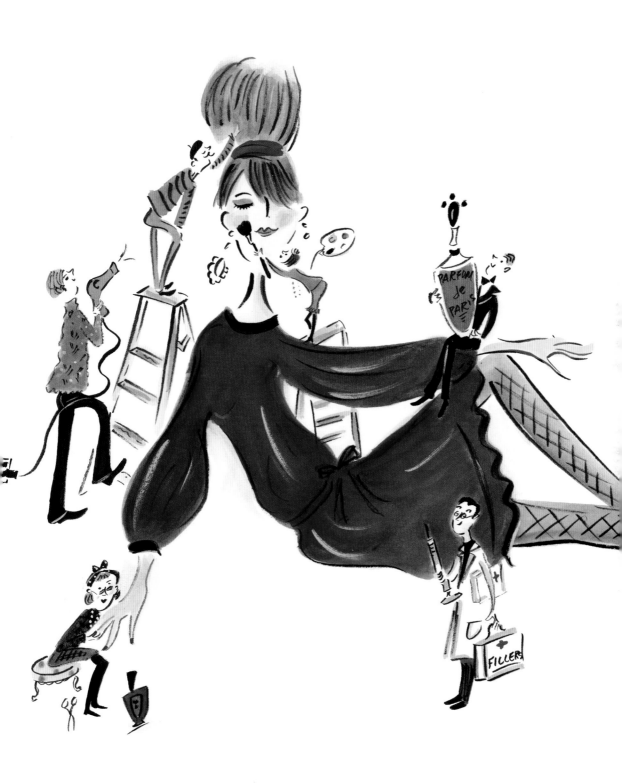

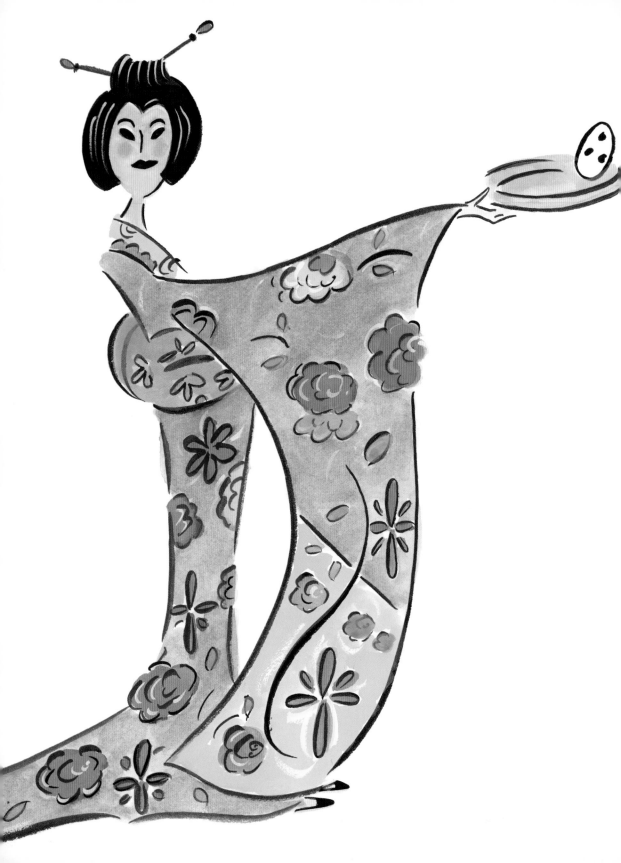

CHAPTER ONE

WABI-SABI

the perfection of imperfection

YEARS AGO, WHEN I WAS TRAVELING THROUGH JAPAN, I MET ISSEY MIYAKE, THE ICONIC JAPANESE DESIGNER KNOWN FOR HIS MODERN FASHION DESIGNS. Since he was a man of distinctly refined tastes, I jumped at the chance to visit the local spa he recommended. The spa was known for its simple beauty, its organic architectural style (an artful abundance of wood and rock), and its elegant proprietor—a beautiful woman in her fifties. It was here, during a traditional tea ceremony, that she exposed me to the aesthetic of *Wabi-Sabi*, a Japanese concept that celebrates the beauty of imperfection, especially as it relates to the changes experienced with the passage of time. With quiet ritual, she presented a spare bamboo tray laden with an array of irregular-shaped wooden bowls wearing a sheen of time-earned patinas, and old cracked pottery that had been fired with subtle, earth-toned glazes. Together, they presented a beautiful picture of restraint, purity, and color that was a reflection of time's passage. *Wabi-Sabi*, the proprietor explained, was the acknowledgment and respect for imperfection (the

Wabi-Sabi: It is the opposite of trying too hard, and it is understanding the power and seduction of imperfection.

cracks in the pottery), the aesthetic of imperfect beauty (the irregular bowls), and the important notion of honoring time and simplicity (the patinas and glazes). *Wabi-Sabi*: It is the opposite of trying too hard, and it is understanding the power and seduction of imperfection—the beauty of an egg with spots, a seashell with water marks, and, like the beautiful spa owner, a woman with laugh lines. It is the perfection of imperfection, a profound reminder that beauty is best found in its least complex form.

How does this philosophy apply to us? Let me start by sharing an anecdote . . .

When I worked with Ralph Lauren, he told me that the girl he designs for is the one in the convertible with the top down, her hair and clothes blowing in the wind.

I've never forgotten this and I've carried that girl, that image with me, into my womanhood. The French say, *"Elle est bien dans sa peau"*—she is comfortable in her own skin, like the girl in the convertible, not concerned that her hair and makeup look perfect. This is true *Wabi-Sabi*.

We each want to capture that totally natural and carefree girl inside us—the one who is completely at ease with herself and her look at any age. We all know the woman who tries too hard, does too much, and becomes enslaved by the latest trends. She's the woman in the spin class who is so made up that she can't break a sweat, or the woman at the beach with false eyelashes and bright-blue eye shadow, or the woman shopping for groceries wearing lip liner in one color and lipstick in another, or so much lip gloss that she can barely move her mouth when she speaks. She's the woman you don't really ever get to know because her hair, makeup, and clothes enter the room before she does—not a strand of hair, not an eyelash, not a stitch out of place. She has lost that girl.

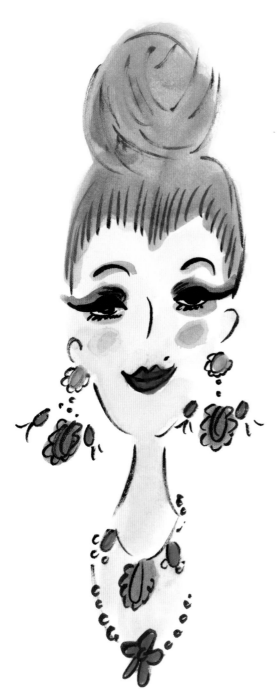

The beautiful older Japanese woman in the spa and the girl in the convertible rule my beauty routine. They are the personification of beauty in its simplest form, not sepa-

She's the woman you don't really ever get to know because her hair, makeup, and clothes enter the room before she does.

rated by age, but joined by their engagement in living and appreciating life as it happens, and the vigorous acceptance of imperfection.

So in light of this, you might ask: How much do I have to worry on the beach, on the ski slope, on a blustery day? How do I strike the balance between not enough and too much control over my appearance? And: Can I still look natural and be fashionable at the same time, young in spirit but not over-the-top trendy? The answer: of course. It's all about *Wabi-Sabi*. And this chapter is about how to make it work for you. Here are the overarching truths:

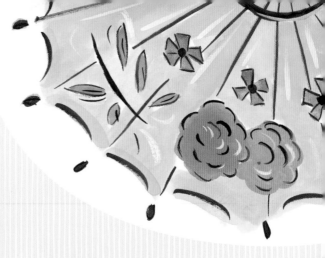

1 LET GO OF PERFECTION

This is a tough concept, because we've all been brought up to strive for perfection in one way or another. But the truth is that embracing your "flaws" makes you more beautiful, more noticeable, more accessible, more real. How attractive! These are the qualities that come with experience and awareness. Learn to love the bump in your nose, the asymmetry of your eyes, your uneven mouth, your freckles. Learn to love what you consider your flaws.

2 BEWARE OF TRENDS

While I do not subscribe to the rigid rules that many women's magazines like to dictate about how to look good at every age, there certainly are trends you can carry with confidence at age twenty that simply don't work when you're over fifty. Most makeup trends are targeted to women eighteen to forty years old. And that should be your first clue that beauty companies are not thinking about us with the products they market. Furthermore, much of the beauty content we read in fashion magazines is provided by these beauty companies. So beware: What looks good on the model in the magazine may not look good on you. Beware of screaming color. Beware of raccoon eyes. Beware of the latest yellow eye shadow. Beware of heavy eyeliner. Beware of frosted eye and cheek color. Beware of high-gloss lips. Beware of overpenciled, overarched brows. Master the difference between trend "aware" and trend "beware." Just be aware that these looks have been bought and sold by major corporations, but only you can own your personal beauty.

3 DON'T TRY TOO HARD

Let's face it: Wearing heavy makeup when you're over fifty—especially in everyday settings, like the woman at the spin class, the beach, or the supermarket—is as off-putting as seeing short-shorts on jiggly thighs. So the first rule of thumb is to beware of being sold the "short-shorts" of beauty. Remember, department store

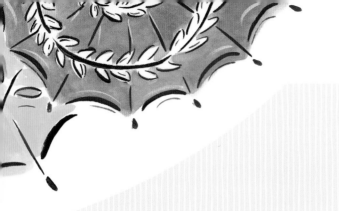

that glittery teal eye shadow. And that matte fuchsia lipstick. Oh, and those colored mascaras, too. Refuse all those inappropriate and cringe-worthy trends of our younger years!

cosmetics "experts" get a commission for selling you stuff that you don't need and stuff that is frequently not appropriate. How can you avoid this? First, take a good look at yourself in the mirror and review recent photographs of yourself. Consider what you see. Is your favorite lipstick too harsh? Your eye makeup too heavy? Is that color that the beauty advisor with the ring in her nose at the MAC counter sold you too garish for you? Take an overall assessment: Are you wearing too much powder and paint? Decide what to get rid of. If you're having a hard time with this, pay special attention to Chapter 2 and don't be afraid to consult with a trusted friend whose taste you admire about what works and what doesn't in your makeup kit.

When in doubt, remember what the late Diana Vreeland, the legendary editor of *Vogue* magazine, once said: "Elegance is refusal." And I'll add my own two cents: "Fear of change is for old ladies!" So retire

4 HIGH MAINTENANCE HAS TO GO

When it comes to makeup, your routine should be effortless. It shouldn't take more than ten minutes. No, I am not kidding. If it takes much more than that, rethink and re-edit your regimen. This book will help you do that.

And when it comes to cosmetic quick fixes like fillers, please take my advice and don't become a junkie. If Botox is the cocaine of the upper face, then Restylane is the crack of the lower face. Be judicious in what you choose to do. And beware of the Botox/filler parties that closely resemble the Tupperware parties your mother went to. Only now there is a doctor or a nurse with an arsenal of botulism and perhaps some bovine fillers waiting to freeze your face, not the leftovers, at an expense far greater than a set of microwave-safe plastic containers. Just a little reminder: Crow's feet and laugh lines equal a life well lived.

5 SAY "SAYONARA" TO HARSH LINES

And a tough and angry disposition equals a life *not* well lived. And it shows up as scowl lines on your face. And there's nothing pretty about that. The same principle applies to makeup—harsh lines have to go! Check your eyeliner, lip liner, contour lines, and eyebrow pencils. If any of these products are creating sharp lines and hard edges on your face, they should be banished from your makeup case. You need cosmetics that blend, blend, blend. The best look is soft like the wind in the hair of the girl in the convertible. Remember: Makeup is an expression of who you are—not who you were, not who you thought you'd be, and certainly not what the media tells us we should be. Who you are is actually much better. Trust me.

6 DON'T BREAK THE BANK

If you add up all the dough you've ever forked out for beauty products that you either didn't need or didn't use or ended up throwing away, you could probably buy that convertible that inspired Ralph Lauren (or take a trip to that spa in Japan), and you'd still probably have enough money left over for a Birkin bag. To look good, you don't need to spend a lot. It's fine to shell out for certain special "pricey" pieces—but head straight to the drugstore to economize on the rest. You'll find recommendations of how to do this in every chapter.

7 BE PROUD OF WHO YOU REALLY ARE

Do you ever wonder what Dolly Parton looks like under the pounds of makeup and all that blonde, cotton-candy hair? Wouldn't her voice still be as great without it? Wouldn't she still be as funny and clever without it? Wouldn't she still write the most heartfelt and perceptive songs without it? Wouldn't her guitar sound just as good without her long nails? When people say they love her because she's so real I know what they mean, but I always wonder why she needs to pile on the paint, camouflaging her natural beauty. Maybe it's cultural, maybe it's the fans, maybe it's the media. Maybe it's her inner mirror. Does she really *see* herself in all her brilliance? Dolly Parton is not alone. Many other women fall prey to this, despite their innate talent and beauty.

8 LOVE YOUR LINES, YOU'VE EARNED THEM

You're not twenty anymore, and that's a good thing, so I'll say it again: Your lines are what make your face interesting. They are lines of *expression*. Think Diane Keaton in the movie *Something's Gotta Give* (rent it!). She shows us that being beautiful has nothing to do with age or lines or spots. In the end, she, not the younger babe, gets the guy. Remember, you're not twenty anymore and that's a good thing. Accept your laugh lines, laugh about them, and use them to your advantage.

accept your laugh lines . . .

So what does all of this mean? It means appreciating where we are in life, the experiences we've had, and the changes we've made—or those that have been made for us. It's harnessing all of that energy to express the beauty we possess and how to make it work for us in everyday life. In fact, it's understanding that beauty has nothing to do with age and everything to do with a comfort zone the years have provided; that our wisdom, experience, and emotional maturity have coalesced into a beauty that provides a precious platform for our physical appearance. We honor who we are and the abundance of our talents by respecting our physical appearance.

At fifty and beyond, *Wabi-Sabi* teaches us to inhabit the beauty that comes effortlessly with age. It is time for *us* to own our face, not Estée Lauder, not Maybelline, not Revlon, not L'Oreal. It's time to release ourselves from slavish devotion to beauty gimmickry.

At this point in our lives, our beauty routine should be more minimal and effortless, and more strategically focused on the right products and the right procedures in the right places. This is a new day, and we're turning the page to a new beauty chapter for ourselves. And this is where I come in . . . read on.

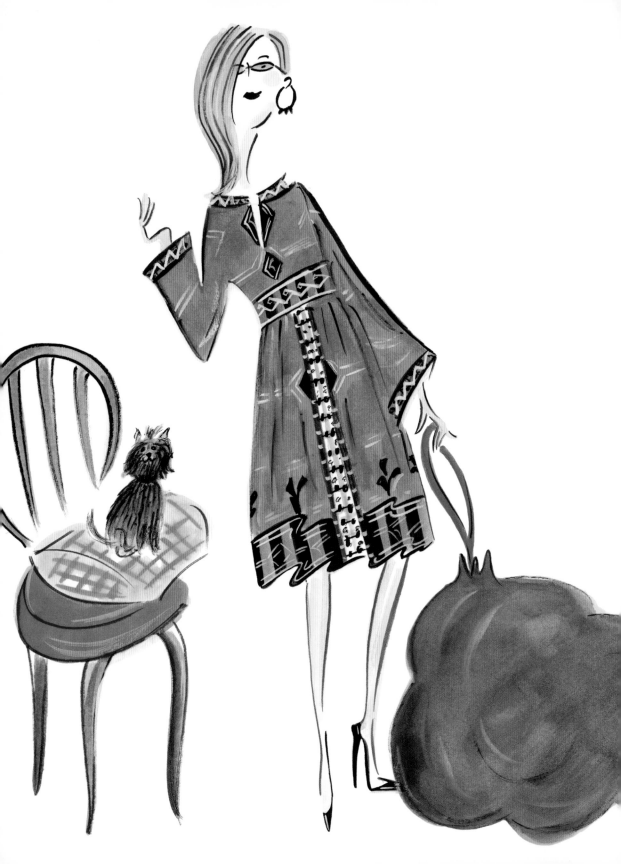

CHAPTER TWO

Out With The Old

clear the shelf and free yourself

BE BRAVE AND TAKE THE FIRST STEP: A FACELIFT. NOW, DON'T GET NERVOUS! IT'S NOT FOR YOU.

It's for your bathroom vanity. By shaving years off your shelves, you'll be left with fresher, healthier beauty products that will enhance your appearance and protect you from the nastier consequences of using old cosmetics. The added beauty of downsizing to the essentials is that you should then be able to tote them easily in a single, well-chosen makeup bag, making storage and retrieval as simple as a one-sided zip.

If you're thinking, *How can I possibly reduce half a dozen drawers and shelves to a single bag?!* I've got news for you. Follow these directions:

1 Get a tall kitchen garbage bag (preferably biodegradable, since the containers you toss will likely be recyclable). If you're at all like me, you will need the big thirty-gallon outdoor garbage bags instead, or maybe even a U-Haul truck!

2 Sweep, dump, or scoop every cosmetic product you've owned longer than one year into that bag. Whatever you do, *don't* stop to debate whether you'll have another chance to wear that sexy red lipstick you bought for New Year's Eve last century, or the shimmery bronzer you bought for your trip to Hawaii three years ago. You won't. *You shouldn't.*

3 Immediately toss the bag(s) into the recycling bin—preferably the one outside—and banish all second thoughts. Congratulations. Now go back inside as fast as you can.

Purging is good. I'm talking about getting rid of all the stuff you don't need—the C-R-A-P that's standing in the way of reclaiming your beauty (and let's face it, your sanity). Chances are, you have a lot of cosmetics that have outlived their expiration date. Keep in mind that the clock starts ticking the moment you open a new tube, wand, bottle, or lipstick, and be aware that natural beauty products have a shorter shelf life because those parabens you've been trying to avoid—the chemicals found in malignant breast tumors that mimic estrogen—were developed to prohibit bacterial growth.

purging is good . . .

Unlike food, cosmetics aren't required to have an expiration date printed on their packaging, so it's up to you to keep track of when you purchased them (see sidebar for specifics about the shelf life of common beauty products). For example, that old tube of opened mascara you've been hoarding for longer than four months is likely laden with bacteria, and there's nothing pretty about a case of pink eye. What about that foundation you've been saving for a rainy day. Is it separating in the bottle? Dump it! Old foundation can clog pores, irritate skin, and cause breakouts. Are your sponges old and torn? Are your powders crumbling? Has that fabulous eye shadow changed color or faded? Do your products look dirty and smell bad? What about all those opened tubes, compacts, and lipsticks that you've had trouble parting with for years?

"Be brutal" is the operative phrase here.

Think they'll come in handy at some point? *Uh uh,* they've gotta go. If you haven't used a cosmetic in six weeks, it's a pretty safe bet you aren't going to use it any time soon. Get rid of it, all of it.

"Be brutal" is the operative phrase here.

I know this might be difficult, especially if you spend more money at Sephora than you do on your monthly mortgage. But do you really want to risk a bad case of middle-age acne, or, worse, a staph infection? I think not.

Ultimately, you just don't need all those products to begin with. Say buh-bye to all of it and hello to a very important beauty truth:

BEAUTY TRUTH:

Beauty comes from within . . .
a very small makeup bag!

---

the bare necessities

This chapter is about having access to your everyday beauty essentials—not excess; just enough to fill a small and practical makeup pouch, and nothing more. Think of it as a diet program for beauty products—like Weight Watchers for cosmetics, and the following items are the essential "food" groups:

FOUNDATION OR TINTED MOISTURIZER

Because these products give you the color and luminosity that menopause steals. The right one makes you look dewy, fresh, and glowing. The wrong one makes you look like Casper the Friendly Ghost. Choose carefully (see Chapter 5 for more about foundation).

CHEEK COLOR

Because this pick-me-up product takes you from dull to vibrant in five seconds or less. It's like a latte for your face.

LIP LINER

Because it restores fullness and shape to your lips and reins in runaway color that loves to migrate into the vertical lines above your upper lip.

LIPSTICK

Because it restores the creamy texture and volume of youthful lips. (An inconvenient truth: Gooey lip gloss is for Dallas Cowboys cheerleaders and your teenage daughter. Toss it immediately.)

MASCARA

Because the eyes are the most expressive part of the face, which may be why this is the classic "desert island" makeup item of choice (assuming there is someone else on the island and you already have sunscreen).

EYELINER

Because it enhances the natural beauty of the eye. It can even reshape the eye.

Now let's talk about organization, because almost as important as what products you keep on hand is how you organize and store them, what you tote them in when you're on the go, and which cosmetics products you should keep at work for a quick day-to-evening transition without a stop at home.

vital reserves

If your cosmetics storage area is anything like mine, it's so full that you likely have to body-slam the cabinet door shut and hold it for a few seconds before gently letting go, hoping it doesn't burst open and the contents come tumbling out. Yep, I *am* the one who could use a few thirty-gallon garbage bags! So let's do this together.

First, we're only going to save a few pieces from each of the essential "food" groups listed above. For example, assuming their expiration window is still open, keep two foundations or tinted moisturizers (for seasonal changes), two or three blushers to work with seasonal and lipstick changes, three lip liners to match your lipstick colors, three of your favorite lipsticks in a range of colors, two mascaras (one waterproof), and two eyeliners.

Now where do we put all this? Space is the defining factor. Most of us keep our cosmetics in the bathroom medicine cabinet, but this is the worst place to store cosmetics because it is warm and damp, which speeds up the deterioration of the product. Instead, keep your products in a cool dry place removed from moisture and light (for starters, consider a shelf in your clothing or linen closet). To get even more longevity from your products, place your cosmetics

> To get even more longevity from your products, place your cosmetics in a plastic box with a tight lid and store them in the refrigerator.

in a plastic box with a tight lid and store them in the refrigerator. Don't worry, this will not affect the texture or application properties of your cosmetics; just give the products time to warm to room temperature before using.

As for what type of container to store them in, see the list below for some tried-and-true suggestions:

HANGING ORGANIZER WITH CLEAR POCKETS

These affordable organizers can be hung on the back of a closet or bathroom door, and they come in a wide range of sizes and styles. Check out the selection at Bed, Bath and Beyond (www.bedbathandbeyond.com).

STACKABLE STORAGE BOXES

Preferably transparent, with removable drawers. The Container Store (www.containerstore.com) offers a wide range of sizes and styles, including those hard-to-find smaller acrylic organizers and caddies with separators that can be most useful in tight spaces.

TACKLE BOX OR TRAIN CASE

Check out www.target.com for the Soho or Caboodles brand of cosmetic cases. Like tackle boxes, they unfold, revealing several levels of built-in storage cubbies.

DRAWER ORGANIZERS

If you're storing cosmetics in a drawer, try a flatware organizer for simplicity. The Container Store is another great place to look for drawer organizers in various shapes and sizes.

SHOEBOX

Yes, I mean it. In the absence of all of the above, you can go with an old-fashioned sturdy shoebox—or upgrade to a pretty box with a lid. Simply separate the products into clear plastic baggies. Repurposed cups, canisters, and pencil holders also make great receptacles for brushes or eye and lip pencils. Look at it this way—you're saving money *and* reducing your carbon footprint at the same time.

With these few pieces stored in an easily accessible place, there'll be peace in your closet and a feeling of well-being in your soul. Say, *aaah . . .*

say, aaah . . .

office supplies

If you work outside the home, it's always handy to have a stash of the right makeup at the office for impromptu after-work outings or just to freshen up before a staff meeting, client appointment, or power lunch. A little cosmetic pick-me-up during the work day will help boost your confidence and enhance first impressions. Keep in your desk drawer a small, preferably transparent, container or standard makeup pouch—anything that fits neatly at your work station and is accessible—and fill it with the basics and then some. Here are three simple steps to fleshing out your workplace backup kit:

1   Keep on hand cleansing towelettes, a facial moisturizer, a travel-size pack of tissues, and a mini magnifying mirror (if you can find a small one with a suction-cup back, all the better—you can stick it on any flat surface, allowing both hands to be free).

2   Next, choose the lipstick and lip liner that looks best for evening, and buy an extra one of each to go into your office kit. Add an eye shadow for a smidge of drama, and transfer some of your foundation or tinted moisturizer into a travel-size container (available in most chain drugstores). A friend of mine keeps hers in a contact lens case—small enough to fit in a pocket, and it keeps the makeup fresh. (Note: The foundation formula and the plastic container may not be compatible; should the product start to change color or consistency, toss and switch to a small glass container.)

3   Now add your tools. Be sure to keep your sponges, Q-tips, sharpeners, and makeup brushes in a separate container or clean baggie to help limit the buildup of bacteria.

All of this should take up no more than half a desk drawer. A great fashion tip that I learned from my first boss—*Mademoiselle* magazine editor Nonnie Moore, who rarely went home before attending glamorous events and dinners—was to tuck an all-purpose evening clutch in the drawer, in the event of any postwork festivities.

on the go

So now it's time to move on to your hand-bag, possibly the most important makeup carrier you own. What do you take with you on a daily basis? Do you toss your makeup into your purse alongside your keys, change, and wallet? Or do you keep it in a nice zip-pered pouch? Your makeup should be kept together in a bag or pouch so you don't have to hunt around the bottom of your purse for your lipstick—or worse, have your makeup leak all over the inside of your bag.

One of the chic-est women I know—a well-respected former *Vogue* magazine edi-tor, Jade Hobson, only uses Ziploc bags to contain her cosmetics because she prefers the ease of seeing the particular product she wants. When the bags get dirty or smudged, she replaces them. If you prefer an actual makeup pouch, look for these impor-tant qualities: small and washable, with a dependable closure.

You can find affordable, sturdy, easy-to-clean makeup bags online, or you can often snag higher-end bags at a fraction of the cost at discount department stores like TJ Maxx or Ross, or from vintage resale shops. Check out the following websites for worthy brands that offer quality bags below $100.

www.toryburch.com

www.katespade.com

www.lesportsac.com

www.sephora.com

For those interested in a little splurge (and no doubt you've earned it!), let me introduce you to a few high-end designer makeup bags that will not only stand the test of time and wear but are so well made that each tiny detail conveys their iconic ele-gance, luxury, and craftsmanship. And, not to be ignored, they pack a lot of purse power (your friends will notice when you take it out of your bag)! Years of experience have shown me that quality really does count, and these three designer classic bags have it in spades:

quality really does count . . .

THE PRADA BLACK NYLON ZIPPERED BAG

Choose the smallest size and make good use of the inner zip pocket. It's lightweight, indestructible, and the zipper is totally reliable. This cosmetic pouch is thoroughly modern and a true favorite of beauty editors.

THE LOUIS VUITTON MONOGRAM MAKEUP TROUSSE

Made of high-quality coated canvas, it's sturdy, rarely shows makeup stains or handbag scuffs, wipes down quickly with a damp cloth, and the monogram design reeks of vintage luxury worthy of nothing less than *Downton Abbey*.

THE HENRI BENDEL POUCH

Made of signature brown and white vinyl-coated cotton twill, its plastic coating makes it impervious to damage, spills, and leaks. This classic makeup carrier is the go-to bag for many makeup artists.

While these designer makeup cases are a big splurge item, investing in them is a great "cost per wear" (CPW) strategy, since they will last you a lifetime and never lose their luxurious presence and appeal.

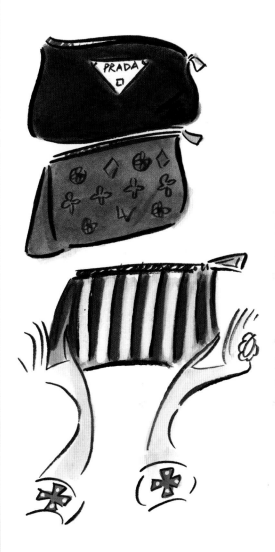

buyer beware

Have you ever fallen prey to the GWP (that's "Gift with Purchase" in makeup speak)? You know, those makeup bags that come "free" when you buy a product from a beauty company? Those little totes brimming with mini makeup products, like mascara, lipsticks, and eye shadows? If you have, don't beat yourself up, we've all been taken in by the Gift with Purchase promotion. Once you read this, you'll think twice about succumbing again. Here's the true scoop on how the

But the GWP is really not a gift, and it's not free, because you can't get it without making a purchase!

GWPs work: It's the cosmetics company's way of luring you to their counter. You make a purchase, and only then are you rewarded with your Gift with Purchase. You may have intended to purchase only one product, but you'll likely go home with three, since the beauty advisors, who are paid on commission, are trained to not let you escape with less than three products. But the GWP is really not a gift, and it's not free, because

you can't get it without making a purchase! To add insult to injury, the cosmetic pouch is so cheaply made, it can't take a lot of wear and tear (all is not lost—you can use it to store tampons, Q-tips, or cotton balls in your desk drawer). Further, it's filled with tiny product samples with colors and formulas that are often not right for you.

Bottom line, the manufacturers want you to sample and get hooked on these products because they can produce them in huge quantities at a low cost.

Cosmetic companies and retailers spend millions of dollars on full-page newspaper adds, online banner ads, and in-store promotions to advertise these GWPs. Picture the conversation in the marketing department of these companies during a brainstorming session on how to design and sell the GWPs. You know what, never mind—you don't need to imagine the conversation because, as a beauty executive, I've heard hundreds of them. They all go something like this: "The pouch is too expensive! Get rid of the buckle, get rid of the

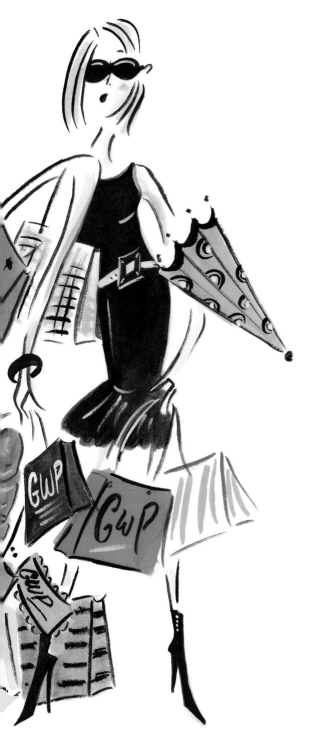

pockets, get rid of the zipper, and use a snap instead. Can't we find a cheaper fabric? Can't we make it in China? How can we produce this pouch for $1.00 instead of $1.10?" It's all about cheap, cheap, cheap.

Still not convinced? Just ask yourself how many of these products and pouches you have actually used, or saved with the intention of regifting them, only to have them take up space in your drawers and cabinets for months, even years, never to see the light of day until you clean out the closet and put them in that thirty-gallon garbage bag.

Bravo to all the hoarders of the world who can bring themselves to take the first step: Toss and make room!

The Gift with Purchase shenanigans were started by Estée Lauder years ago as a sampling vehicle, and much of the cosmetics industry followed that lead because it created enormous sales. That said, beauty companies are increasingly pulling away from these promotions because they are not realizing the same return on investment they once did (too much competition, and loss of interest by the consumer), but nobody's willing to ride out the drop in sales that would come as a result of dropping GWP entirely. So, dear buyer, beware of strangers bearing "gifts" (with purchase).

So here are some questions to ask yourself as you are flinging "gifts" and purchases into the trash bag:

1 How many seasons ago did I buy this product? In other words, is it a "fad" color? (Probably.) Should I be wearing a "fad" color in the first place? (No way.)

2 How many times have I worn this? If the answer is never, time to gift it to someone who can, like the local women's shelter—if the products have never been opened. (Virgin olive oil is great, virgin makeup is wasting valuable counter space.)

3 Am I just hanging onto it because I'm feeling guilty for spending so much? (You might want to ask your wardrobe this one, too.)

4 Am I holding on to an empty bottle thinking I might reuse it? (That's why God invented recycling bins.)

5 Would my daughter wear this? (See also: Would my mother wear this?)

6 Why did I buy this in the first place? Who talked me into it? (If it was one of your friends, maybe you need to toss them, too.)

7 And the key question . . . do I really need all this crap? (No, no, NO!)

Toss and
don't look
back.

Face it: It's impossible to mentally keep track of when you purchased which products. Short of creating an Excel spreadsheet, here are some tips to keep you clued in to when your products are out of date:

- Label your products. Stickers are colorful reminders of expiration dates, so you can easily label a specific product by its particular shelf life. You can find waterproof stickers for this purpose at www.beautyalert.biz.

- Download the Beauty Alert! app, which keeps track of your cosmetics. It will notify you when they expire.

- Use a Sharpie pen to write down the purchase date on the product container itself.

- Put a "toss" reminder on your calendar.

Prolong the life of your products and prevent contamination by doing the following:

- Never borrow a product that someone else has used.

- Sharpen lip and eyeliner pencils after each use to remove moisture-causing bacteria, which contaminate the pencil.

- Choose makeup products in sealed pump containers. This allows you to dispense the product without introducing new bacteria.

- Periodically wipe lipsticks with alcohol wipes.

- Do not store makeup in the bathroom if you can help it. Keep it in a cool, dry place to ensure its longevity.

When should you replace your makeup? See the list below for the general rule of thumb on how frequently you should toss and replace standard cosmetics once they've been unsealed. Natural beauty products have a shorter shelf-life since they're free of preservatives, so they should be replaced every six months (except for mascara or unless the product package indicates otherwise).

- **MASCARA:** Every three months

- **LIPSTICK/LIP GLOSS:** Every twelve months

- **EYE SHADOW:** Every twelve months

- **PENCILS FOR EYES AND LIPS:** Every six months

- **LIQUID FOUNDATIONS, CONCEALERS, HIGHLIGHTERS, AND TINTED MOISTURIZERS:** Every six months

- **POWDERED FOUNDATION, BLUSH, HIGHLIGHTERS, AND BRONZERS:** Every twelve months

- **CREAM BLUSH:** Every six months

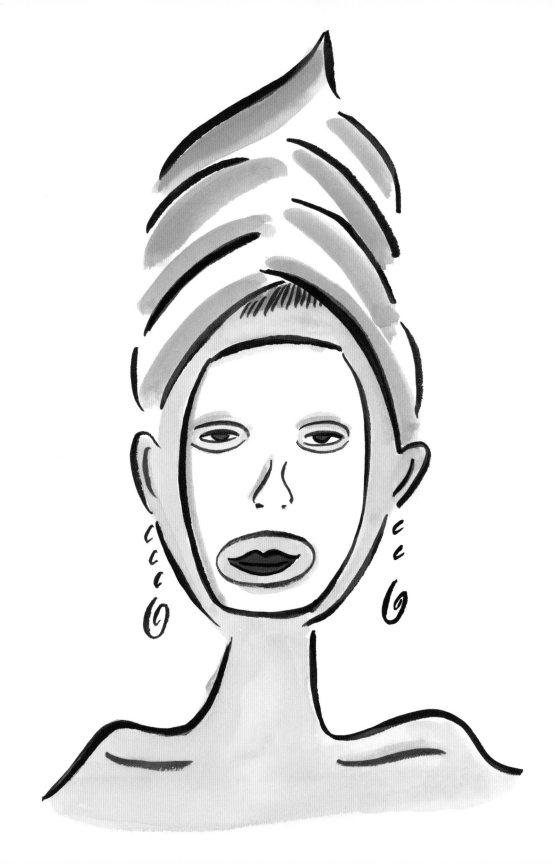

CHAPTER THREE

Skincare

getting clear on product help vs. hype

THERE ARE MORE ANTIAGING PRODUCTS OUT THERE THAN GEORGE CLOONEY HAS EX-GIRLFRIENDS. THE PROBLEM? FEW OF THEM ACTUALLY DELIVER.

The skincare market may be one of the few that has embraced women over fifty with open arms—at least, in theory. The beauty companies are preying on our insecurities about aging rather than acknowledging how damn good we already look. I mean, do we really believe this season's "new" miracle ingredient will make us look ten years younger? (Wait, do you also believe in unicorns?) We might be savvy enough to know when we're getting duped, but even the smartest among us will be surprised at some of the beauty-industry marketing she-nanigans. But first a reality check.

Sure, you've accumulated a few more laugh lines, perhaps even a new age spot or two, but the changes are more than just skin deep. You've also changed *physiologically,* and that means a whole new set of rules for how your skin behaves. That's right, I'm about to invoke the "M" word: menopause. (If you're not quite there yet, you will be, so read on anyway.)

Without getting too technical, I'll just tell you that our skin becomes drier, thin-ner, and less elastic at menopause because of the natural lowering of estrogen levels (unless you're taking hormone replacement therapy, which has its definite downsides—ask your doctor). The decrease in this key hormone can result in a number of beauty bummers (including less hair on our heads and more on our chinny-chin-chins). For now, however, let's focus on the effect it has on our skin. There is a direct link between lower estrogen levels and reduced collagen and skin elasticity, thickness, and strength. Gone is the perky plumpness you used to take for granted. Your skin is probably look-ing and feeling a lot more parched now, and when you pinch the back of your hand, it probably stays pinched for far longer than it used to. Yep, this stinks. But if we're hon-est and open in talking about it, we can take the necessary steps to deal with these effects and start to get in touch with our new and improved beauty routine instead. The first step is to know the difference between skin-care products that help you offset these age-related tempests and skincare products that merely offset your bank account.

brand beware

Beauty counters are brimming with slick-looking moisturizers, serums, peels, oils, masks, eye creams, lotions, and night treat-ments that promise to combat wrinkles, crow's feet, bags, and sags. The options are seemingly endless and the choices can be overwhelming. And unlike the "beauty con-sultants" at cosmetics counters who work on commission and are trained to parrot their company's product press releases, I will actually tell you the truth: Smoke and mirrors abound.

Having spent a big chunk of my career in the high-tech research and development laboratories of some of the world's most prominent beauty companies, I can share an industry scoop that most women don't know. Major beauty corporations own or license several brands in a wide range of price points. The Estée Lauder Companies have Bobbi Brown, Clinique, Tom Ford, La Mer, MAC, Estée Lauder, Smashbox, and a myriad of other brands. The L'Oreal Group has Maybelline, L'Oreal Paris, Lancôme, Ralph Lauren, Kiehl's, La Roche-Posay, Redken, Matrix, Essie, and others. Procter and Gamble owns CoverGirl, Max Factor, Olay, SK-II, to name a few. And Coty owns Philosophy, Sally Hansen, Rimmel, and OPI. This information is on the Internet, but it's certainly not broadcast by the individual brands that often compete against each other.

In my career as a beauty editor, I saw the industry's top beauty brands present new skincare offerings every season, and I quickly learned to connect the dots. Basically, one research lab in each corporation fuels the technology development and creates an ingredient that is widely used across many of their brands. They get away with it by using different scientific-sounding names for the ingredient, and they carefully wordsmith the claims for each brand so they don't sound exactly the same. So while L'Oreal Paris would introduce a product with glamorous packaging, a space-age name with ingredient X, and an

> The first step is to know the difference between skincare products that help you offset these age-related tempests and skincare products that merely offset your bank account.

ad campaign featuring a celebrity spokesperson, Lancôme might introduce virtually the same product with ingredient X "respun" with a chic French name, different luxury packaging, and a slightly different claim for essentially the same ingredient. The only real difference? The price. L'Oreal Paris is sold in drugstores and Lancôme is sold in department stores as a higher-end brand. In the end, it's all pretty much the same stuff. For example, a few years ago, Lancôme's big launch of the season was Genifique, a "youth-activating concentrate" stemming from the production of genes. Similarly, a year after this launch, L'Oreal

Paris introduced Youth Code Serum Intense that touts a breakthrough using "gene science"—get the connection?

And even more shocking, did you know that big corporations compete to buy or license a "hot" ingredient or technology very often from the same two or three independent laboratories, and then claim that ingredient as their own creation?

And did you also know that the moment one of these companies creates a new "it" product that garners beauty awards and reaps high retail sales, the rest of these beauty companies waste no time copying it and getting their own version to market, posthaste? All of the above brings us to another . . .

BEAUTY TRUTH:

The tubes from Target will probably work just as well as the bottles from Barneys.

Save your money for a guilty pleasure and invest in skin care the way you would stocks: cautiously, wisely, and well-informed. I'll be your broker.

tricky wordsmithing

When it comes to touting a product's benefits, beauty companies have developed hocus-pocus phrases best left to noncommittal boyfriends to market their promises to unsuspecting consumers.

Do phrases like "may help to diminish" or "results may vary" sound familiar? This is where you need to be extra vigilant. Nontransparent words like "may" express only the *possibility* that the claim may be true. These "promises" or claims are vague for a reason. Companies use the word *may,* as in "may improve" and "may lift" to ensure that they are not caught making false claims about how the product works, which would leave them open to lawsuits based on false advertising. How about promises like, "refill wrinkles in just one hour"—sound tempting? Keep your refills to a glass of Chardonnay! The key word in that phrase is "refill" versus "remove forever," because the reality is, it's temporary and it doesn't say how much your wrinkles will be refilled or that they will go away. You may see some short-term improvement in skin because of hydrating ingredients that soften and "plump" the look of stubborn wrinkles, but the wrinkles will still be there in one hour and tomorrow. This is not necessarily a bad thing, but it's important to be clued in about

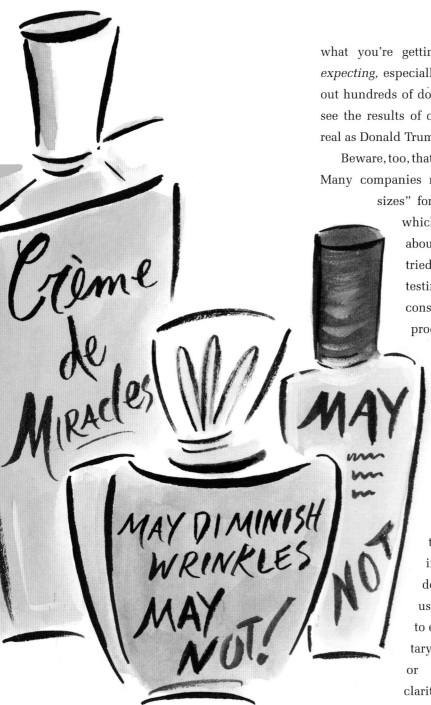

what you're getting versus what you're *expecting,* especially when you're shelling out hundreds of dollars a month hoping to see the results of claims that are about as real as Donald Trump's comb over.

Beware, too, that little asterisk symbol (*). Many companies refer to "small sample sizes" for their research groups, which might suggest that about one hundred women tried it, when in fact the testing group may have only consisted of twenty-five product users. You don't know how the research was conducted, so don't fall prey to this. These claims give the impression that they were conducted using the most rigorous of scientific methods, but often these studies are lacking in real supporting evidence. Beauty companies use this punctuation mark to endorse vague commentary like "in a clinical study" or "instantly improves clarity." Follow the asterisk, and you'll see qualifying statements for claims such as "69 percent clinically measured improvement in overall aging signs after 12 weeks." Sounds promising, right? But read the mice type associated with that asterisk (in the magazine gutter), and you'll read the *context* of that claim: "*12 week

Brace yourself: Like the promises politicians make during the campaign season, many of these product promises just aren't going to happen.

clinical test conducted on 32 women aged 26–64." Not a big sample size, and certainly not a sample size reflective of the target audience. I mean, just how many women were over fifty and how many were dewy-skinned twentysomethings? There is nothing remotely scientific about it. Then why even include it on the packaging? Because this little punctuation mark is intended to protect the company from being accused of misguiding the consumer with unfounded or unsupportable claims, and the company is hedging their bets that you won't bother to read the fine type, and, if you do, that it

won't make much of an impression because it still sounds clinical. The same goes for phrases like "dermatologist-tested," which marketers like to use to coax you into thinking a dermatologist hand-picked that product, tested it, and gave it a blessing, when in reality all it means is that a product has reached a certain level of safety in the company that's making the claim, but, since the cosmetics industry regulates itself, there are no industry-wide standards for product testing. And don't be lured in by clinical-sounding language like "Our studies show . . ." Don't get excited that 95 percent of women found positive results. All this means is that 95 percent of the women tested could simply have noticed a difference and liked a product, which isn't the same as 95 percent seeing an improvement that matched the product's claims, like an actual reduction in wrinkles!

Believe me, the research and development labs in these corporations are smart and know how to establish their tests for the appearance of outstanding results. Brace yourself: Like the promises politicians make during the campaign season, many of these product promises just aren't going to happen. But don't be discouraged! Some products actually *do* deliver, and we'll get to that soon.

be wary of endorsements

There are other ways beauty companies mislead consumers in their effort to sell us their products. When it comes to endorsements, for example, beauty editor "favorites" are not always true favorites. Believe me, I know, because I was once the beauty editor for *Vogue*. Here's the scoop: Before I began work on the editorial content for each new issue, I was given a "must list" from my publisher, whose job it was to bring in advertising dollars—which, for the uninitiated, is how all magazines pay for their overhead costs, including staff salaries. As you can imagine, there's a lot of pressure from big advertisers to promote their products, so this list included the products and companies I must mention on the pages of the magazine, based on the number of advertising pages a particular company has bought for the issue or for the year. The silent quid pro quo was basically "no ticket, no laundry," or no editorial mention, no advertising. Sad but true—not all favorites *are* favorites and journalistic integrity is not always exactly pure when it comes to editorial content— let's leave it at that—just be aware that when it comes to "must-have" beauty products, the favorites are often written by editors with fingers crossed behind their backs.

Celebrity endorsements work the same way. The celebrity negotiates a hefty contract (often in the millions of dollars) with a beauty company that requires her to say she uses and loves the product during press events, like product launch parties, store appearances (where it's being sold),

> Just be aware that when it comes to "must-have" beauty products, the favorites are often written by editors with fingers crossed behind their backs.

print advertising, TV commercials, magazine and Internet interviews, and personal appearances on television talk shows. So when you look at Starlet X's skin in the ad and think it's so perfect, remember Photoshop, and, when you hear her praising the product's benefits, remember that she's paid to do so.

And what about skincare brands marketed under the name of a famed dermatologist? Just because a product carries a doctor's name doesn't necessarily mean he created it. Many suppliers (the labs that create and manufacture these formulations) offer "stock" products, similar to a shoe store that has different sizes of the same shoe available in the stock room. Sometimes a scent is changed, a color is adjusted, or an ingredient is added to the base formula, but, basically, the dermatologist often slaps a label on it and calls it his or her own. The products that actually have been developed by doctors usually are aesthetically pleasing and offer a new ingredient, but the truth is that, even with those, nothing new has been added to the equation. Remember that although doctors (derms) are involved with patients' skin issues, they are not scientists (the people who have made the breakthroughs). In most cases, he/she'll sell these products to patients as a follow-up measure to "enhance" or "help prolong" the benefits of the treatment she's just received, and their products are a profit center for them.

But despite all this skincare strife, there are things you can do, buy, and use (and *not* use) that really will enhance the appearance of your skin. Here's some real advice about what works and what tanks, and what I consider to be the most effective, investment-worthy skincare ingredients and products available to you.

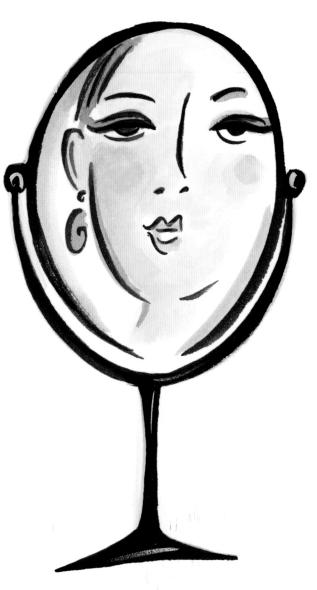

SLEEP

FACT: OUR SKIN CELLS REGENERATE WHILE WE SLEEP!

Get that "beauty" sleep (seven or eight hours nightly does it for most of us) whenever you can for healthy-looking skin. A good night's sleep does make a difference to our skin, as it repairs and restores itself while we rest. Lack of sleep makes the skin appear dull and lifeless and accentuates dark circles under the eyes. The Debbie Downer fact is that menopause is often accompanied by restless nights (sorry to report this) and those sweet dreams can be interrupted by hot flashes and night sweats. But the good news is that we can do something about promoting more restful nights.

It took me a while to get the hang of it, but here are a few tips I've learned for all you sleeping beauties:

- No caffeine for six hours before bedtime
- Eating a light and early dinner regularly
- Going to bed at the same time every night
- Limit alcohol intake to one glass of wine daily
- Regular exercise

Forget sleep aids. I gave those up when a friend emailed me back with question marks in response to an incomprehensible email I'd sent him in the middle of the night, which I had no recollection of doing! No thank you to those little devils. They went into the thirty-gallon bags with my expired cosmetics.

EXERCISE

FACT: INCREASED BLOOD FLOW AND CIRCULATION NOURISHES SKIN CELLS.

It will also chase away those nasty free radicals (see the following page) that damage good healthy skin. Exercise eases stress and therefore we can often fall asleep more easily—one big happy circle of health that feeds into the heart, lungs, and SKIN. Make it a regular routine four or five times weekly, alternating disciplines of aerobic, muscle, and stretching. I also am a great believer in squeezing it in when it presents itself to me (e.g., a flight or two of stairs or a fast walk to a destination—when alone I always walk fast).

SUNSCREENS

FACT: SUN DAMAGE IS THE #1 CAUSE OF WRINKLES.

There is no advice I can offer you that is more important than this: Use a sunscreen! It is the lion at the gate of healthy, even-toned, beautiful skin. Do not leave home without it. Rain, sleet, snow, or hale—not just when you're on the beach—use a sunscreen *every day*, everywhere. Be sure it's "broad-spectrum" (titanium dioxide, zinc oxide, or Parsol 1789), which blocks the wrinkle-causing UVA rays and the burn- and cancer-causing UVB rays. Use at least an SPF 30, but don't waste your money on anything higher than an SPF 50, since there's little evidence that higher SPFs provide more protective benefits. This is a skincare item that can be purchased quite inexpensively just about anywhere, from drugstores to sporting good stores.

Here are a few **Best Bets:**
- Aveeno Protect & Hydrate Lotion Sunscreen with Broad Spectrum SPF 50 For Face
- La Roche-Posay Anthelios SX Daily Moisturizer Cream with Sunscreen
- Shiseido Urban Environment Oil-Free UV Protector Broad Spectrum SPF 42

ANTIOXIDANTS

FACT: FREE RADICALS ATTACK HEALTHY SKIN CELLS AND BREAK DOWN COLLAGEN, CAUSING DULL SKIN AND WRINKLES.

Antioxidants do battle with these nasty molecules, which are produced by pollution, stress, alcohol, cigarettes, and sun. Antioxidants are found in berries, pomegranates, grapes, and foods rich in Vitamin C and E, green tea and even chocolate(!), to give a few examples. Additionally, topical use of antioxidants in the form of an oil, serum, or cream has proven effective relating to natural and synthetic light damage.

Some **Best Bets** worth considering:
- SkinCeuticals CE Ferulic
- Elizabeth Arden PREVAGE Anti-Aging Daily Serum
- La Roche-Posay Active C Anti-Wrinkle Concentrate

RETINOIDS

FACT: THE ONLY PROVEN ANTIAGING COMPOUND THAT REDUCES LINES AND WRINKLES.

Retinoids increase cell turnover and stimulate collagen renewal, which is the support structure that gives skin a firmer look—exactly what our fifty+ skin needs. The most powerful punch comes from prescription strength retinoids, but over-the-counter products will still yield impressive results. Retinoids should only be used at night, as sunlight can inactivate them and there are risks or side effects, like redness and flakiness from exfoliating skin with prescription strength that your doctor can help you manage.

A few **Best Bets** to try:

- RoC Retinol Correxion Deep Wrinkle Serum
- Vichy LiftActiv Retinol HA Night Total Wrinkle Plumping Care
- SkinCeuticals Retinol 1.0 Maximum Strength Refining Night Cream
- Philosophy Miracle Worker

ALPHA HYDROXY ACIDS

FACT: ALPHA HYDROXY ACIDS REMOVE THE TOP LAYERS OF DEAD SKIN CELLS, LEAVING DRY SKIN MORE DEWY AND GLOWING.

Alpha hydroxy acids (derived from food), which are used as a skin exfoliant, are most commonly found in face peels but are also found in a multitude of cosmetics products, from cleansers to moisturizers, and are used as a lower concentrate and more gentle ingredient (as opposed to retinoids). They come in the guise of glycolic acid, lactic acid, citric acid, and other fruit acids. It is best to follow use of these acids with a moisturizing sunscreen since the top layers of the skin are exfoliated and, like retinoids, skin is more photosensitive after using these natural chemicals. Also worth noting, some redness and flaking may occur, but don't be alarmed! This is part of the process. (Warning: Read labels carefully before trying at-home acid peels.)

Here are several **Best Bets** I recommend:

- Dr. Dennis Gross Alpha Beta Peel Original Formula
- Jurlique Fruit Enzyme Exfoliator
- Peter Thomas Roth Un-Wrinkle Peel Pads

SALICYLIC ACID

FACT: SALICYLIC ACID TREATS ACNE BY REDUCING SWELLING AND IRRITATION AND UNBLOCKING SKIN PORES.

Salicylic acid (derived from tree bark) is part of the beta hydroxy family. Both alpha and beta hydroxy acids work by sloughing off dead or damaged skin on the surface of your face, encouraging new, fresh skin to appear. The main difference between the two is that beta hydroxy is oil soluble and can penetrate deeper into the clogged pores to actually break up sebum. Salicylic acid is most effective when dispensed in prescription strength by a dermatologist. It has been proven very effective in treating acne, which many of us still struggle with at menopause. There are several over-the-counter strengths of this substance, but it can often irritate the skin, so it must be used judiciously and only as directed.

If you have menopausal skin eruptions, you might try one of these **Best Bets:**

- La Roche-Posay Effaclar Medicated Gel Cleanser
- Neutrogena Healthy Skin Anti-Wrinkle Anti-Blemish Cleanser
- Vichy Normaderm Triple Action Anti-Acne Hydrating Lotion
- Clinique Acne Solutions Cleansing Foam

SKIN WHITENERS/ AGE SPOT REDUCERS

FACT: SOME PRODUCTS EXIST THAT CAN REDUCE AGE SPOTS AND EVEN OUT THE SKIN'S APPEARANCE, BUT BEWARE OF PRODUCTS CONTAINING HYDRAQUINONE.

Never ever use a skin cream containing this nasty ingredient, which is banned in many countries. Not only can it irritate and damage the surface of the skin, but evidence suggests it can also cause damage at the DNA level. Yes, it does produce results, but at a potentially great cost to your health. There are other products on the market that do not contain hydraquinone and are considered safe. These products require continued use to see a visible difference.

Here are two **Best Bets** worth mentioning:

- Clinique Even Better Dark Spot Corrector
- Garnier Skin Renew Clinical Dark Spot Overnight Peel

MOISTURIZERS

FACT: MOISTURIZERS THAT DO NOT INCLUDE THE PREVIOUSLY MENTIONED INGREDIENTS GIVE A TEMPORARY EFFECT OF PLUMPING UP, LUBRICATING, AND SOFTENING THE SKIN AND RESTORING ITS SUPPLENESS.

The operative word here is "temporary." To retain this effect, a moisturizer must be used at least twice a day, every day. There is nothing appealing about dry, lifeless skin no matter what our age, so it's a good idea to use one. Hyaluronic acid is a popular ingredient in moisturizers because it draws moisture from the air and holds up to 1,000 times its weight in water. This ingredient does NOT eliminate wrinkles when used topically, and it does NOT penetrate the outer layers of the skin. Hyaluronic acid provides only temporary dry skin relief, but, for the sake of comfort and the look and feel of more supple skin, should be used. Some other moisturizing ingredients that are effective emollients are high-quality oils like camellia, macadamia, rosehip, and argan.

Here are some **Best Bets,** effective classics, and newer oils:

Classics

- CeraVe AM Facial Moisturizing Lotion (my dermatologist's favorite)
- Olay Regenerist Micro-Sculpting Cream Moisturizer
- Crème de La Mer
- L'Oréal Paris Revitalift Volume Filler Re-Volumizing Daily Moisturizer

Oils

- Rodin Olio Lusso
- Trilogy Rosehip Oil
- Josie Maran Argan Oil

CLEANSERS

FACT: IT'S IMPORTANT TO WASH YOUR FACE BEFORE BED EVERY NIGHT.

Never, ever hit the pillow without clearing your face of the day's makeup, grit, and grime. What we want at this stage of the game is a no-frills, gentle cleanser that does not dry out the face.

Three very simple, good **Best Bets** are:
- Cetaphil Gentle Skin Cleanser
- Dove Beauty Bar
- CeraVe Foaming Facial Cleanser

THE MAIN POINT: Forget night creams, forget toners, forget eye creams, forget neck creams, forget collagen, forget firming creams, forget lifting creams, forget décolleté creams, and forget super expensive creams. Use a moisturizer instead, and stick with the list above. These are the ingredients or products that will move the needle on your skin. Accept the reality that there are no magic bullets, no instant face lifts.

Just ask your dermatologist (if he or she is not contracted as a spokesperson for a cosmetic company).

Read on and be happy to know that help is on the way, that a few simple skincare products, some strategic cosmetic staples and tips combined with a sensible lifestyle, can do more to enhance the appearance of your face than any "miracle" cream, lotion, or potion.

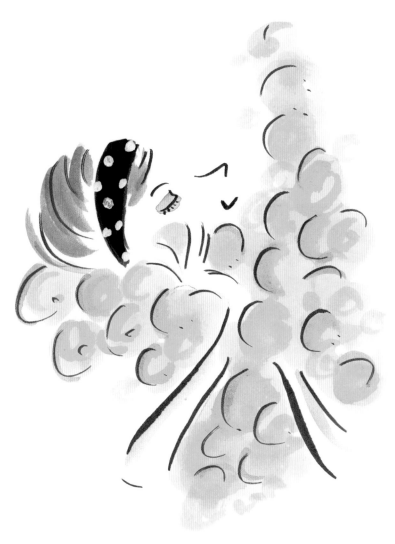

THE PROS AND CONS OF HRT

Menopause, like adolescence, is a fact of life, but it doesn't mean we have to embrace the less glamorous side of aging. I should know; menopause hit me hard and fast in my early forties. As my estrogen levels dipped, so did the collagen in my skin. As my testosterone (the male hormone) increased, so did the hair on my face. And my once-prized dewiness? Done. I was not going down without a fight. My weapon? Hormone Replacement Therapy (HRT). While it is currently the most common way to temper the toll that aging takes on our youthful selves, it does have a dark side—not unlike a menopausal mood swing.

I asked Dr. Michelle Warren, director for Columbia University's Center for Menopause, Hormonal Disorders, and Women's Health, to weigh in on the risks and benefits.

"There are many good things about HRT," she said, adding that while the positive impact on the appearance and elasticity of our skin is very individual, "it generally improves." It also helps combat the suite of symptoms that plague us—from hot flashes and moodiness to painful intercourse and insomnia—and may help offset bone loss and heart disease. Additionally, a recent study she conducted showed that women on HRT were generally happier and more satisfied professionally. But, she cautioned, there are well-documented risks, including blood clots, stroke, and breast cancer (striking 1 in 1,000 women per year).

The takeaway here?

"[The choice] is very individual," she said. Like any health-related decision, it's important to consult very closely with your doctor, since all women's needs and bodies are different.

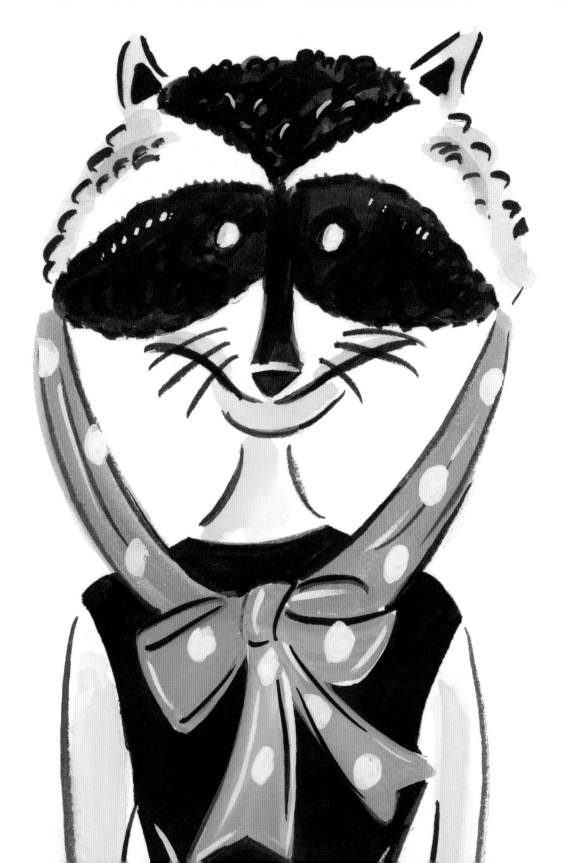

CHAPTER FOUR

Eliminate & Illuminate

concealer, primer, highlighter

REMEMBER WHEN YOU THOUGHT EVERY ACTRESS AND MODEL YOU SAW ON THE PAGES OF GLOSSY MAGAZINES HAD FLAWLESS SKIN? WE'RE A LOT SMARTER NOW THAT WE KNOW ABOUT AIRBRUSHING AND PHOTOSHOP.

And it certainly doesn't hurt that beauty bloggers, gossip columns, news outlets, celebrities, and outspoken models themselves are patrolling beauty companies for truth in advertising—and then calling them out on their practices. Remember when Jezebel.com exposed Faith Hill's unretouched (and still beautiful) photo that appeared on the cover of Redbook? Or when TheCut.com showed a before-and-after shot of an Ann Taylor catalog, and the fashion and beauty industry stopped dead in its tracks?

We no longer have to feel stressed about not looking anything like those celebrities and models who, "au naturel," don't look anything like themselves. We've already established that we *do* want to look like our-

We're older and wiser, so instead of wishing to be who we were, we're going to embrace the adventure of who we can become.

selves, only better, and by now we should know this book isn't about reclaiming your youth or looking like a model. If you've learned one thing from me so far, I hope it's that aging is *not* a flaw. We're older and wiser, so instead of wishing to be who we *were,* we're going to embrace the adventure of who we can *become.* How? By investing in some minimal cosmetic wizardry via a few simple products, which you will thank me for telling you about later.

But before I reveal this surprisingly simple beauty alchemy, let me share a true story from my magazine days that will give you a laugh *and* a deep appreciation for the handful of cosmetics effective at camouflaging imperfections when necessary:

We were shooting a very big star for the cover of a magazine, and my editor-in-chief insisted the actress look fresh, clean, and entirely natural. This was after the celebrity's very messy and very public divorce, and after she had thrown herself into her work, shooting back-to-back movies. By the time this woman got to us, she looked like she needed a spa week instead of a photo shoot. We had hired a makeup artist whose skills I had admired but I had not yet worked with. The star and the makeup artist met, and within minutes I could cut the tension with a machete. The big dispute: The makeup artist refused to use a concealer to cover the actress's undereye circles, which were darker than the espresso she was drinking. The star abruptly excused herself and disappeared into the ladies room. When she did not return to the set after twenty minutes, I went to the ladies room to see what was wrong—frankly, I was worried she'd blown off the shoot and fled to her car and driver waiting downstairs. But there I found her, in front of the mirror holding a powdered doughnut from the catering table. She wasn't sneaking junk food, she was, believe it or not, delicately dabbing the powdered sugar from the doughnut under her eyes to cover her dark circles! I saved her any additional angst and immediately dismissed the arrogant makeup "divo," dispatched my assistant to pick up the star's favorite concealer, and applied it myself. She stepped in front of the camera and a beautiful magazine cover was created. She looked fabulous, and very natural, but I learned a great lesson from her panicked moment: Always have a concealer on hand.

For women of a certain age—*our* certain age—there is an almighty trio that's going to keep you looking better than ever:

CONCEALER
Think of this as your magic wand. It makes all bad things disappear.

PRIMER
Think of this as Spanx for your face.

HIGHLIGHTER
Your lightening rod, attracting light to key places on your face.

This chapter will teach you how to use all of the above to master the fine art of "concealing," coupled with the even more refined art of revealing, and how to cosmetically cope with lines, wrinkles, circles, and spots so that you get that fresh, youthful look.

get that fresh, youthful look . . .

concealer

Let me repeat a fundamental lesson from a previous chapter. Modern makeup means concealing more by using less. This is especially true for women our age. What exactly do I mean by this? Here's an example: We've all seen people who've used a heavy spackle-type concealer in a shade much lighter than their foundation to hide their dark circles. That never works. Unfortunately, they end up looking like a raccoon. Not a good look, unless it's Halloween. Which brings me to an important . . .

BEAUTY TRUTH:

Your foundation and concealer must be the same color.

Did you record that? It's so important. Read on for facts and tips that will help you master the blend and conceal.

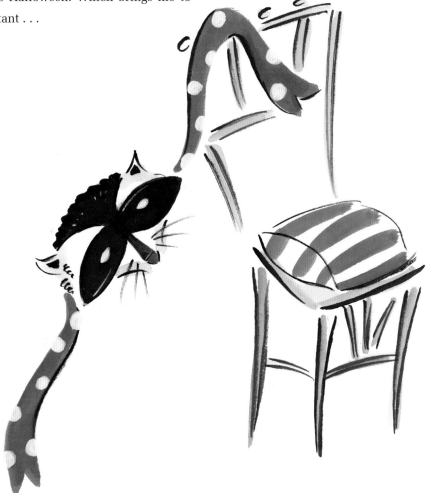

FOR YOUR EYES ONLY

If you have dark circles under your eyes, the worst thing you can do is apply a thick, dry, and pasty concealer in a lighter shade than your foundation! It will only make you look worse because it will emphasize wrinkles and bags. Here's the right way to handle dark circles, in three simple steps:

1 Start by applying foundation to your entire face.

2 Next, layer a heavier dose of foundation over your dark circles. Use a small, stiff, flat brush and build up carefully to an adequate coverage. If this doesn't do the trick, move to a concealer. I repeat, of the same color.

3 Apply your concealer with a light hand, layering it thinly over your foundation and "patting" it in place with the same small, stiff, flat brush (or use your ring finger or a high-quality silk sponge, "patting" with gentle pressure). Concealer for this area of the face should be moist and malleable (liquid or creamy texture).

NOTE: Make sure the concealer blends with your foundation *all the way down to your cheekbones*, and, if necessary, apply a bit more of your foundation on top. Pat, pat, pat away until both are seamless.

Here are a few **Best Bets** for undereye concealers that really work:

- Clé de Peau Beauté Concealer (expensive but worth it)

- Lancôme Waterproof Effacernes

- Maybelline New York Cover Stick Correcter Concealer

- Almay Wake-Up Undereye Concealer

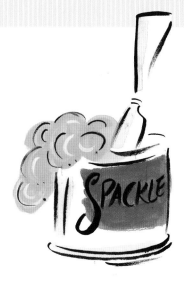

REIGNING IN ROGUE SKIN

Our skin suffers countless assaults, from acne, blemishes, birthmarks, and spider veins around the nose, to undereye dark circles and brown spots. You and I probably have at least one of the above. I am always waging war on my brown spots (a.k.a., age spots) and blemishes, and this is when a different consistency of concealer is required. However, I underscore once again how critical it is that your concealer matches your foundation (I know you don't want to look like the Halloween raccoon with freckles, as this concealer requires a spot application). With this type of concealer, I prefer to apply my foundation first (but see below—concealer first is fine, too).

When covering these difficult areas, the best tools for applying concealer are a clean Q-tip, a clean synthetic washable brush, or a clean synthetic washable sponge. I emphasize *clean*; it's best not to use your germ-spreading fingertips, especially when dealing with acne or blemishes. The consistency of your foundation-matching concealer for these special needs should be more opaque, not very malleable, and less creamy, since you want it to stay without moving on the spot you are covering. A more solid, dryish texture works best and is usually found in a pot. Follow the three-step method for flawless coverage:

1 Target with precision and apply the concealer, then wait until it dries.

2 If the blemish is still visible, apply again; wait for the concealer to settle.

3 Reapply a thin layer of foundation to the touched-up areas.

target with precision . . .

You might wonder which comes first, the chicken or the egg? Foundation or concealer? The truth is, either is fine in this case. My preference is foundation first. When applying foundation first, apply the foundation, then dot concealer on the spots where you need extra coverage. But I encourage you to experiment; try applying concealer first. You might discover you don't need foundation, or need only a little to even out your skin tone. Try both ways and see which works best for you.

CONCEALER SPOTS THAT YOU SHOULD KNOW ABOUT BUT PROBABLY DON'T:

- Inner dark corners of the eyes for brightness (especially good for Mediterranean and Latina origins)

- Outer corner of the eyes for an upward illusion

- Either side of the mouth for an upward illusion

By now, you've learned that you probably need two different kinds of concealers for best results: a creamy, moisturizing one for dark undereye circles, and a drier textured one for dark spots, acne/pimples, and redness.

This is my list of concealer **Best Bets** for those "special needs" areas:

- Dermablend Smooth Liquid Camo Concealer

- Cinema Secrets Ultimate Foundation (use as concealer)

- Laura Mercier Secret Camouflage

And a couple of **Best Bet** zit-fighting concealers with salicylic acid:

- Neutrogena Skin-Clearing Blemish Concealer

- Murad Acne Treatment Concealer

primer

Now let's talk about Spanx—for the face, that is. You know Spanx's "power panties"? I couldn't exist without them; the über camouflage they provide for my protruding belly and fulsome hips. Well, girls, turn your attention to a power primer. After the diet program for your makeup bag I spoke about in Chapter 2, this would be the first few ounces I would

> Take it from me, a good primer makes your foundation or tinted moisturizer roll on more smoothly, filling in wrinkles, lines, and pores. It also covers most dark circles, and makes your foundation last longer.

"put on." Yes, it's another step (swap the powder for this). No, I didn't wear it when I was younger, but, after my skin started to change, primer and I formed a codependent relationship. The key is to test-drive several different types. You need to find the one that's going to work well with your foundation. Primers can be very drying, so look for a hydrating texture (unless you are going to use it on your oily T-zone), and forego the colored ones (green, orange, and lavender) and the gels. Take it from me, a good primer makes your foundation or tinted moisturizer roll on more smoothly, filling in wrinkles, lines, and pores. It also covers most dark circles, and makes your foundation last longer. Apply primer after you've moisturized and sun-protected your skin. It's like waterproofing your skin; it holds in the moisture and prepares your skin for the next layer—tinted moisturizer or foundation. Primers come with SPFs built in and some can be worn alone without makeup.

My **Best Bets** for a range of skin types:

- Clarins Instant Smooth Perfecting Touch

- Laura Mercier Foundation Primer—Hydrating

- Sunday Riley Effortless Breathable Tinted Primer (can be worn alone)

- MAC Prep + Prime Face Protect Lotion SPF 50

- NYC New York Color Smooth Skin Perfecting Primer

- Benefit Cosmetics The POREfessional Face Primer

- L'Oréal Paris Studio Secret™ Professional Magic Perfecting Base

highlighter

Welcome to the land of Tinker Bell, fairy dust, and happy thoughts. I don't know about you, but I could use all three. Highlighters, used subtly, can transport us to Never Never Land. In my book, that's the land of less wrinkles, less gray pallor, less thin lips, and less droopy eyes. We "never never" want to have those issues. Highlighters can diminish features like receding chins and wide noses, and accentuate features like high cheekbones. The secret of highlighters is this: They use light to draw attention to features we want to accentuate and deflect attention from spots we want to diminish—like receding chins, droopy eyes, or a wide nose. Don't underestimate the magic lurking in petite swipes of this versatile product when used in just the right places.

There are many different types of highlighters: sticks, creams, cake powders, loose powders, and liquids. And there are just as many colors and levels of shimmer and glitter. I stick to creams because I find them subtle and easy to control. The color I prefer is a golden or a natural skin tone, with a very low level of shimmer. Highlighters were made to highlight the areas the sun naturally spotlights, so be sure to keep it natural.

> Don't underestimate the magic lurking in petite swipes of this versatile product when used in just the right places.

Avoid at all cost the pearly-white consistencies because they look fake, noticeable, and vaguely stripperish. The rule here is that your highlighter should not be visible. The look we are going for is a good healthy shine and glow where we need it.

a good healthy shine and glow . . .

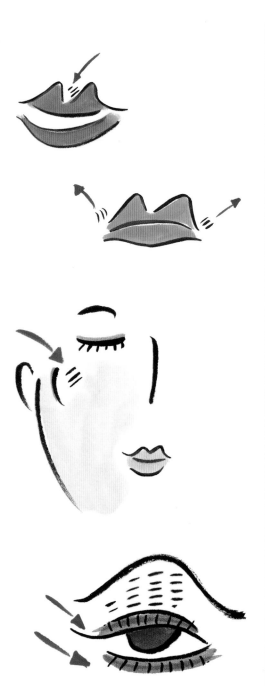

Here are my tried and true tips for how to use highlighter to accentuate or downplay elements of your face:

- Your highlighter has to be lighter than your foundation by at least two shades.

- Apply all highlighter with your finger and blend with patting motion.

- Use for the illusion of a fuller mouth (our lips can start to thin out and lose volume) by applying highlighter to the Cupid's bow (the area between the peaks of the upper lip).

- To avoid a downturned unhappy look to the mouth, dab and blend a small swipe of highlighter at the outer edges of the upper lip at the side of the mouth (concealer can also do this trick).

- After you've applied blush (to the apple of the cheek), dab and pat highlighter across the top of the cheekbone for a luminous, youthful look.

- To emphasize eyes, dab and blend under the arch of the brow. I often work it down on to the lid. There is no need for shadow afterward, just some smudgy dark eyeliner along the upper and lower lash lines. (This tip also helps if your brows make you look angry, disapproving, or tired.)

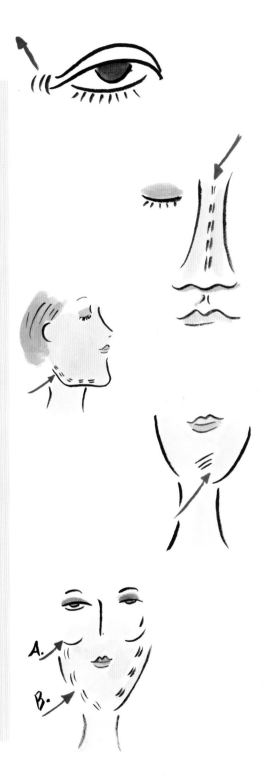

- To avoid drooping eyes, dab and pat a tiny amount of highlighter on the outer edges of the eyes at the side of the upper lids (same idea as the outer edges of the mouth for a slight lift illusion).

- For a wide nose, dab and blend down the center of the nose, starting at the bridge and stopping where nostrils begin to widen.

- For a slackening jaw or jowls, dab and blend along the jawbone, starting where the jowls begin and working your way back.

- For a receding chin, dab and blend a swipe on the middle of the chin.

- For a narrow face, before applying foundation, dab and blend highlighter from (A) the top of the cheekbone (the part closest to the ear) down to (B) the top side of the jawbone. If highlighter disappears, dab and blend on top of the foundation. For a wide face, use a darker shade of foundation or concealer rather than a highlighter.

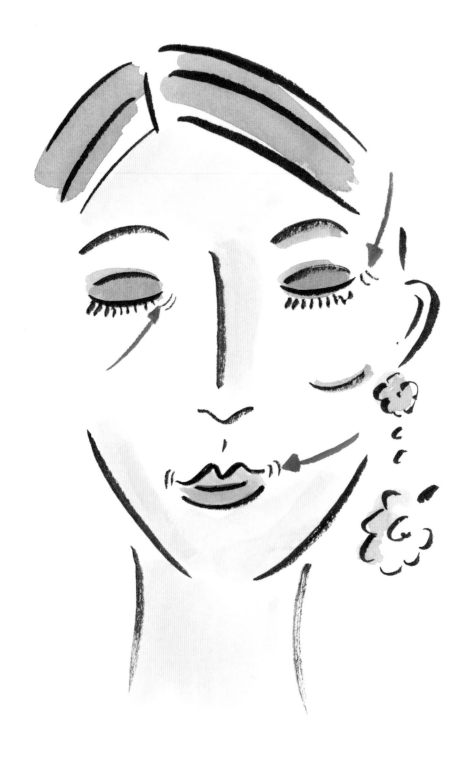

I repeat, a good highlighter will not and should not "read" shimmer in any kind of light. Its purpose is to attract light and to highlight the areas that show you off to your best advantage. Highlighter can be one of the most effective purchases you will ever make, but be very cautious. It's just like overdone plastic surgery: Used inappropriately, this can make you look weird. If you don't know what I mean, think Joan Rivers.

Here are some highlighters worth highlighting:

- Clinique Up-Lighting Liquid Illuminator

- e.l.f. Essential Shimmering Facial Whip

- Yves Saint Laurent Touche Eclat

- L'Oreal Studio Secrets Professional Magic Lumi Highlighting Concealer

- Dior Skinflash Radiance Booster Pen

Concealer, primer, and highlighter, affordable antiaging products with real benefits, are the tools that give us the vision to reimagine ourselves. I am seduced by the magic of their effects and the transformation that comes with the mastery of their use. Here's the lowdown: For the absolute best results, tackle one feature at a time.

The trick to conceal more is to use less product. No circles, spots, or acne? Dump the concealer. No splotchy skin? Ditch the primer. You get the gist. Use the trial and error system to discover what and how much works uniquely for you. And believe in change. That's why you're reading this book. The best news? Unlike more drastic and lasting measures, Kleenex, Q-tips, and cleanser wipe it all off, enabling you to experiment, redraw, and reinvent again without stress.

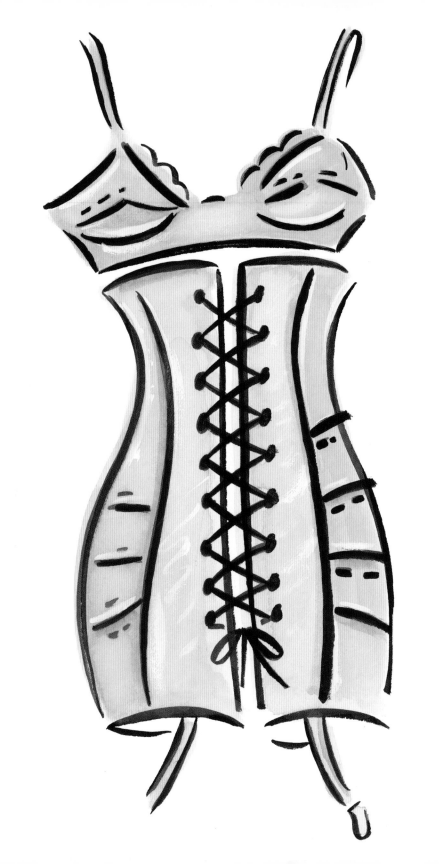

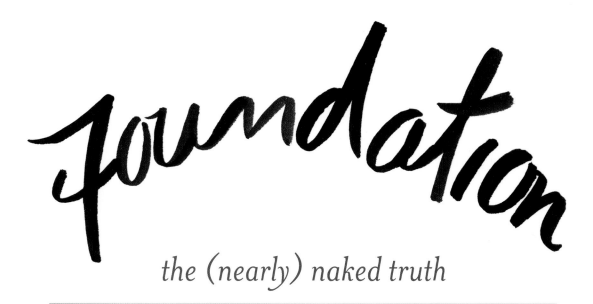

CHAPTER FIVE

Foundation

the (nearly) naked truth

I HATE THE F-WORD—FOUNDATION, THAT IS. IT EVOKES THE CONSTRICTING GIRDLES I USED TO SEE IN MY MOTHER'S UNDERWEAR DRAWER. AND THE WORD BASE . . . WELL, IT SOUNDS JUST BASE. CANVAS ISN'T MUCH BETTER.

Is your makeup routine really in the same league as those reusable bags you bring to Whole Foods? Do you really want your face to look like a blank slate: boring, lifeless, and perfect? And anyway, who needs perfect at a time in our lives when we don't want to hold back? We want to be engaging, seductive, vibrant, alive, sexy, and free—anything but blank and perfect. Yes, this chapter is about . . . okay . . . foundation, but there's nothing base about it. Here's the truth. As much as I'm a proponent of all things natural, I don't think foundation is optional. In fact, foundation is almost mandatory; it's the single most important weapon in your cosmetic arsenal. Think of it this way, you know how you're

Well, think of foundation as the perfect white T-shirt of makeup— it's the crucial anchor piece around which you can build the rest of your look.

always on the hunt for that perfect white tee? The one that's clean, smooth, lightweight, doesn't pill, and looks as good under your favorite jacket as it does with a pair of jeans? Well, think of foundation as the perfect white T-shirt of makeup—it's the crucial anchor piece around which you can build the rest of your look. I'm going to tell you how to find the foundation equivalent of your dream tee, but the key to success here is to shed your fear of showing your actual skin. Yes, this sounds counterintuitive, but it will make perfect sense, trust me. Read on and see.

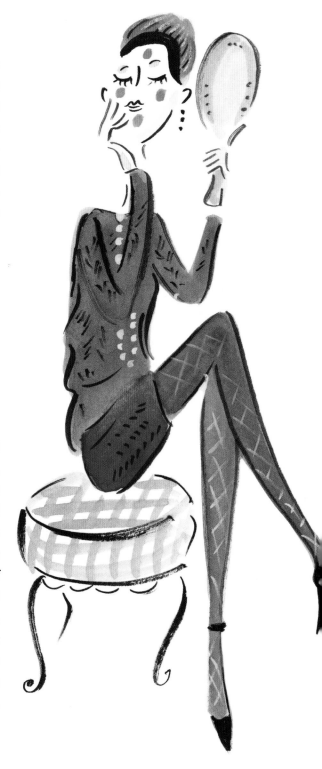

less is more

Here's a beauty trith will real face value; commit this to memory: Revealing the right parts of your skin makes you look fresh and beautiful. Attempting to hide the "wrong" parts of your skin makes you look old. And when I say "old," I mean crypt-keeper old. Thick, pasty foundation will make you look dead. And you know the matte look that magazines insist is so chic? That stuff is great—if you're a sixteen-year-old Ukranian model. Oh wait; you're a real woman? Then toss out those bottles of cement, pronto.

Here's how my less-is-more makeup mantra took root. When I was a beauty editor, I was periodically summoned for tea to the office of the iconic Mrs. Estée Lauder, where she'd introduce the company's new color palette for that particular season. The tea always started out the same way. "Why doesn't a pretty girl like you wear makeup?" (I never told her I was wearing a full face of artfully applied neutral shades.) "Here," she would say, "let me show you how to do something with your looks." Out came that season's palette. And there was no exit possible—you didn't say no to Mrs. Lauder.

While tea with the legendary Mrs. Lauder was always entertaining, she never really sold me on her "more, more, more" approach to makeup; by the time she finished my "makeover," I wouldn't have been able to pick myself out of a police lineup. Even so, I would thank her profusely, promise to consider the colors for upcoming stories in the magazine, and head straight for the nearest ladies room, where I'd scrub and scrub until I recognized myself again, then surreptitiously make my way to the elevator, hoping she wouldn't catch me on the way out.

For me, those visits were an early lesson in what I didn't think worked for modern women: thick, skin-smothering foundation layered under a palette of brights. What does work is finding the right foundation, using it where needed, and warming it up with a little color.

Let's get started.

finding cover

Your mission is to discover a foundation that makes every day a good skin day. The key is finding a formula and shade that blends with your complexion perfectly. In other words, your "skin soul mate."

Finding the right foundation takes time. But don't worry, you can strike foundation gold at almost any point on the price spectrum. This isn't about trading up or trading down on the cost spectrum, it's about Cinderella trying on the glass slipper and finding just the right fit. This perfect fit may requite a splurge, but think of it this way: There is no cosmetic investment that is more important than your face. Of course, there's expensive and then there's stratospheric. For instance, as I write this, you can nab one of Laura Mercier's much-beloved tinted moisturizers for under $50, or splurge on a liquid foundation from Sisley for a cool $115. Often, the foundations created by beauty

And sorry to be a big buzzkill, but you need to hear this (again): You can't rely on women's magazines for unbiased advice either.

companies with a primary focus on skincare, such as Sisley, La Prairie, or La Mer, are extremely expensive. The rationale is that they're packed with many of the same pricey ingredients used in their serums, creams, and antiaging products, which in my opinion is utter marketing babble (more on this later).

If, after scouring the market, you've fallen head over heels for a foundation that clocks in at north of $100, there's an easy way to reduce your cost per wear: Use it sparingly, with a sponge, and only where you really need it. Remember, less is more.

Now let's head out of the high-end department store beauty counter and make our way over to the drugstore. But first, read this:

I mentioned in an earlier chapter that the mega-cosmetics companies behind your favorite department store brands might also manufacture far less pricey lines for drugstores and other mass-market outlets. Remember, this is a win-win for the beauty companies—when a product "hits" with the customer, they're able to apply the same technology to all of their brands, saving themselves a bundle in research and development costs. But for you, it often just means that you're paying more for a department store product, like foundation, then you actually need to. In my view, you can find "just as good" foundation in a drugstore.

But cheaper doesn't always mean honest. You know those ad campaigns plastered all over the cosmetic aisles of your local Rite-Aid or Walmart? The ones with your favorite TV star? As an industry insider, I can tell you that celebrities hawking these affordable foundations aren't necessarily even wearing the makeup they're selling! Celebrities provide star power, period. There is no guarantee whatsoever that they actually wear the foundation they're shilling, so, if you're using the actress from *Modern Family* as a gauge for purchase, you might want to rethink your strategy.

And sorry to be a big buzzkill, but you need to hear this (again): You can't rely on women's magazines for unbiased advice either. Beauty advertising basically supports the magazine business, which is why you'll see countless editorial mentions of a large beauty company's products and very few mentioning the small, independent brands; those niche brands don't advertise—they can't afford to—and therefore aren't helping to fund the magazine's bottom line. And often those cool little "indie" brands get snatched up by the big corporations anyway, because it's cheaper and easier to buy innovation, personality, and street cred than create it themselves. For example, MAC and Smashbox, Kiehl's and The Body Shop, once small stand-alone "indie" brands themselves, all have been "acquired" by the big corporations (Estée Lauder and L'Oreal).

All that information may be a bit of a downer, but the upside to all this makeup madness is that there are a few good products for this stage of our lives at the drugstore *and* the department store. Our first course of action is to determine your ideal shade and the best formula and texture for your skin.

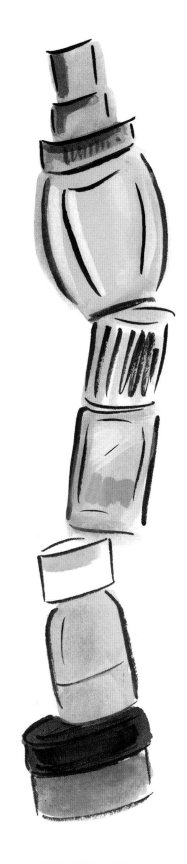

how to shop for the right shade

In your twenties and thirties, the Holy Grail of Hotness is using a foundation that so closely matches your own complexion it all but disappears. But now that we're older, our skin has changed, which means so will the shades that work best for our skin tone. Remember how we touched on menopause in an earlier chapter? Discussing how it changes the elasticity and texture of our skin? Well, it can also change the *color* of

My easy fix to the problem of a fading complexion is to "go for the gold."

our complexion, often making it paler. Since the face is the site of numerous estrogen receptors, any hormonal upset (menopause obviously being the mother of all hormonal upsets) can result in shifts in our complexion, so, after fifty, we typically start to lose the robust color we were once used to seeing. The last thing we want to do is pick a shade that's matchy-matchy with our menopausally challenged skin. (Remember the

pale crypt-keeper? Exactly.) My easy fix to the problem of a fading complexion is to "go for the gold." Simply by shifting into gold and away from those pink-based foundation shades you've been hoarding, you can banish that gray pallor. Foundations with golden (yellow) undertones work magic on your skin. They neutralize any redness and leave your skin looking instantly healthier. Shop for foundation that is a shade darker (two shades, max) than your natural complexion, but decidedly more gold. In other words, run screaming from any rosy tints the salesperson may try to foist on you. They may match your skin color, and they may have looked great on you when you were in your thirties, but that was then and this is now. If you want to look livelier, friskier, and like you're ready to take on the world, gold is the ticket.

Now that you know you need to go gold, you'll still need to find *your* perfect shade for *your* skin tone. It can be a daunting task, for sure. But it's definitely doable.

Apart from made-to-order custom blending (and your options are very limited on this front), how can you get your ideal shade? With all the advances in beauty, you'd think finding the right match would be a snap. It isn't, and one of the reasons involves some inside scoop on the sample situation.

While many of the big cosmetic companies offer a wide range of foundations, they only supply retailers with samples for the three or four best-selling shades. What if the best-selling shades weren't right for your complexion? You wouldn't have the opportunity to take the color home and try it out, so you very well might end up buying a best-selling shade that isn't right for you. It's basically the industry norm to scrimp on samples. But the news isn't all bad. Most department stores (and even a few drugstore chains) have liberal return policies. So if you don't hit a home run the first few times around, don't be shy about making an exchange or asking for a refund. A store that wants your business will be happy to comply. But the goal, of course, is to avoid mistake purchases in the first place. So here are a few quick tips to help you do that:

1 DO AS MUCH ADVANCE-RECON AS POSSIBLE

Before heading to a department store or beauty boutique, pop by a few drugstores (or even one of the "big box" behemoths like Target) and see if you can scrounge up swatch cards or sample-size freebies of shades you think might be right. After testing them at home, you can either head back to the drugstore and buy a full size, or take them with you to use as a shade reference when you're trading up to a pricier brand at a department store like Macy's or at an independent retailer like Sephora. Also, flip through that stack of fashion magazines on your coffee table. These days, some of the mass-market makeup brands advertise by offering a foundation sample that's the equivalent of a perfume scent strip.

2 SHOP WITH A CLEAN FACE

Yes, I know it's scary to expose yourself to the world barefaced, but how else will you be able to sample foundations on the spot? You can mitigate a little bit of that self-consciousness by dressing well, which is not only a great confidence booster, but it's also a sure-fire way to get salespeople to snap to attention.

3 BRING ALONG AN HONEST FRIEND

If you're the type who asks strangers in dressing rooms whether the jeans you've tried on flatter you or not, because, well, you're just not sure and you really need a second opinion, then consider bringing along a trusted friend when you shop for foundation. Be sure it's someone you know will be straight with you, and whose style you admire. Where you see a match they may see a miss.

4 TEST A FEW STRONG SHADE CONTENDERS ON YOUR JAW LINE

Not the back of your hand. Better yet, have the salesperson (if there is one) do it for you. And don't worry, it disappears with one swipe of a makeup-remover towelette. Consider bringing your own wipes, especially if you have sensitive skin, to avoid wearing war paint as you leave the cosmetics counter and head for the shoes.

5 USE THE MAGNIFYING HAND MIRROR TUCKED IN YOUR PURSE

You'll need this when you head outside to play shade detective. The golden shade that looks good in the retailer's fluorescent lighting might look like a topping for hot dogs in daylight. Natural light is the litmus test; make sure any foundation you're considering passes it.

6 BRING A FAVORITE SHADE FROM YOUR BEAUTY STASH

If you're considering trying a new foundation, be sure to bring the one you've been using up until now—as long as the *shade* has been working for you. For example, if your current foundation seems to look dry on your skin and you want to try a product with added moisture and an SPF, having your correct shade on hand will save you a lot of time.

7 DO SOME RESEARCH BEFORE YOU SHOP

Many popular brands have online tools to help you find the right color (L'Oreal Paris even has a new app for that). Or if you know the product and shade, some sites can match it to the equivalent shade in their line.

Natural light
is the
litmus test:
Make sure any
foundation you're
considering
passes it.

One last thought: When you've decided on your shade, you may also want to buy a shade that's one or two shades deeper to accommodate the change of seasons and the months between winter and summer. As the weather begins to change, you can blend the two shades, customizing your palette as you gradually move into the darker shade for the warmer summer weather.

Now that you've got an excellent grasp on the shade you want, the real fun starts: picking a formula that feels great, provides the right degree of coverage, and makes you feel like a million bucks—make that a billion. But to do that, you need to know how to separate the foundation hype from the foundation help. Here's my guideline built on many years of experience:

LABEL LAW 1
AVOID FOUNDATIONS WITH THE FOLLOWING DESCRIPTORS

Anti-Acne

Want an easy way to get dry, cakey, old-looking skin? Apply an anti-acne foundation all over your face. Even if you're experiencing breakouts, I recommend spot-applying an oil-free formula on the problem area only. Beware the "crypt-keeper" look.

Balancing

Aimed at combination skin (i.e., oily in some spots, dry in others), "balancing" foundations seek to level the playing field. But even if parts of your face feel oily at times, your underlying problem is most likely dryness. And for that, you need moisture. Save "balancing" for meditation.

Clarifying

This is just a more ladylike way of saying anti-acne. Most clarifying foundations contain heavy doses of salicylic acid, way too harsh and drying for your "post-M" face.

Long-Wearing

If your goal is a fresh-looking face, this makeup is not for you. Developed primarily for oily types whose foundation tends to slide or melt off quickly, this isn't something you should be looking for. Better to reapply or touch up with the *right* foundation for your skin when and if you need to.

Matte/Mattifying

This could be great if you're twenty-five, but "matte" is makeup code for drying. Trust me, a matte finish is the polar opposite of what you want in a foundation. You're going for glow and radiance.

Oil-Free

Unless you have bonafide adult acne, or a T-zone that's seriously prone to shininess, an oil-free foundation won't do you any favors. Because of hormonal shifts, your skin is likely dry at this stage of the game. Moisture and shine are your friends, so don't fight them.

Powder

A powder foundation looks cakey on dry skin and can be extremely drying (beware of foundations billed as the trendy "mineral powders"). Many powders make claims of hydration, but when you think about it, "hydrating powder" is an oxymoron. At the risk of sounding like a broken record, at our age, we need a *moisturizing* formula.

Self-Adjusting

The theory here is that these wonder brews somehow magically figure out your skin tone and adapt to match it exactly. Don't buy it, literally.

Smart

The kissing cousin of "self-adjusting," smart foundations that go on clear and then miraculously morph into your exact shade are a myth. Until your foundation can tutor your kid for the SATs, don't fall for this ploy.

LABEL LAW 2
BEWARE OF WISHY-WASHY WORDING

I mentioned this before, but it's especially important to remember these slippery words and phrases when purchasing a foundation or tinted moisturizer. They are usually found in the category of "antiaging" foundations, which I don't put a lot of faith in (see the following page). The race is on among beauty companies to lengthen foundation labels with the latest buzz words or ingredients to sound more beneficial than they really are. As with skin care, these phrases are designed to be a block against lawsuits by stating only what a product "might" or "may help" or "appear" to achieve. Avoid these waffle phrases invented to take your money and prey on your insecurities. Companies have made billions on these meaningless claims and ingredients, while covering their corporate asses at the same time. The truth is, the industry uses them to obfuscate the fact that the claim they're making in this antiaging category probably won't do a damn thing for you. Write down this list, carry it with you, and rule out any foundations with the following language:

- "age-defying"
- "appears to diminish"
- "helps to minimize"
- "helps to prevent"
- "improves the look of"
- "may combat"
- "more than smoothing"
- "reduces the look of"
- any phrase that compares the product to cosmetic procedures, such as "lifting," "firming," "antiwrinkle," and "antislackening"

LABEL LAW 3
A CHEAT SHEET OF FIFTY+ BEAUTY-SPEAK

Brightening
Incandescence is the goal of a brightening foundation, and that jibes nicely with the total effect we're after. Just be aware, it can also mean that it contains age-spot diminishers. Read the label carefully—the fewer potentially irritating "treatment" benefits the better.

Dewy
Ah, yes! For all of us, a truly dewy finish is the Holy Grail of foundation textures. Why? Because it means your skin will appear fresh, healthy, and moist. It doesn't get any better than that.

Luminizing
Akin to brightening minus the pigment-diminishing component, luminizing foundations make your skin look like it was lit from within.

Moisturizing
Dry skin craves hydration. End of story.

Radiance
Yet another take on the brightening/luminizing theme. Ergo, a great bet.

Sheer
As long as your complexion is up to the challenge, sheer—the polar opposite of thick, cakey, and masklike—is ideal.

Now that you're armed with discerning knowledge about what beauty-speak to avoid and what to look for in product labeling, it's time to introduce you to the refreshingly broad array of foundation products that work for over-50 skin.

YOU, ONLY BETTER

COMPLEXION-FRIENDLY COVERAGE
FOR FIFTY+ SKIN

Tinted Moisturizer

Hands down, tinted moisturizer is my favorite formula for women of our age. For starters, it helps with menopause-generated dryness, and, just as crucial, it's much sheerer than traditional foundation. Tinted moisturizer is really the only type of foundation product that can be used all over the face without worry of amplifying the aging effect. For day use, try one that has a built-in SPF of at least 15.

My short list of **Best Bets** for a range of skin types:
- Clarins Super Restorative Tinted Cream SPF 20 All Skin Types
- Dr. Hauschka Tinted Day Cream
- Laura Mercier Tinted Moisturizer SPF 20
- NARS Pure Radiant Tinted Moisturizer SPF 30
- Neutrogena Healthy Skin Enhancer Tinted Moisturizer SPF 20
- Philosophy Hope in a Tinted Moisturize
- Sonia Kashuk Radiant + Tinted Moisturizer SPF 15

Alphabet Soup: "BBs," "CCs," "DDs," . . .

Beauty Balms, or BBs, are a hybrid of tinted moisturizer and skin care. The BB cream is most often tinted in one to four shades, with light coverage, and, depending on the brand, may offer sun protection, priming, moisturizing, color correcting, and pore minimizing in a single product. CC stands for "color and correct," and this form contains more pigment and more skincare ingredients than its predecessor, the BB. That means more coverage (like a foundation) and more antiaging claims, such as clarity and reduction of age spots. DD stands for "daily defense" (or dynamic do-all cream). It's reason for being is to include more environmental protection agents, such as sunscreen and antioxidants. Word has it a GG cream is already in the works. Where are we going from here? The newest iterations of these include words like "Miracle," "Blur," and "Magic" in their names to connote some type of transformative experience. Let me repeat: there are no miracles and no magic wands. If some cream miraculously blurs some of your wrinkles, I can assure you it will wash off that night, which is all fine and good as long as you "face" that reality. As far as alphabet soup creams are concerned, I think Philosophy has the right . . . well . . . philosophy. They've named their new "do-all" lotion "A to Z Cream" to hedge their bets and poke a little fun at the whole category.

Consider these **Best Bets:**
- Dior Hydra Life BB Crème
- Estée Lauder Daywear BB Anti-Oxidant Beauty Benefit Crème

- Garnier Miracle Skin Perfector BB Cream
- Chanel CC Cream Complete Correction Sunscreen SPF 50
- Olay CC Cream Total Effects Daily Moisturizer & Touch of Foundation
- Clinique Moisture Surge CC Cream Hydrating Colour Corrector SPF 30
- Philosophy Hope in a Jar A to Z Cream

Liquid Foundation

I'm happy to report that liquid foundations have come a long way since the spackle days of yore. Several glide on seamlessly, delivering sheer coverage that feels virtually weightless. Still, there's no reason to coat your face from stem to stern. Rather, opt for a very light hand on the face, with a slightly heavier application around the nose, cheeks, and chin to cancel out redness.

Check out these **Best Bets:**
- Boots No.7 Lifting and Luminate Foundation
- Giorgio Armani Beauty Luminous Silk Foundation
- Maybelline Instant Age Rewind Radiant Firming Makeup
- Shiseido Radiant Lifting Foundation

Cream Foundations

I love cream foundations because they give great coverage, you need very little to see a visible difference on your skin (great "cost per wear" benefit), they blend easily, have adjustable coverage, and, best of all, you can mix it with your tinted moisturizer (which I do).

My short list of **Best Bets:**
- Chantecaille Future Skin The Foundation Perfect Finish Creamy Formula
- Laura Mercier Crème Smooth Foundation
- Maybelline New York Dream Smooth Mousse

Whipped Foundation

These foundations look and feel great. They offer super aerated, lightweight, smooth coverage that has the look and feel of whipped cream and the ease of application of a liquid foundation.

A couple worth considering:
- Elizabeth Arden Flawless Finish Sponge-On Cream Makeup
- Lancôme Miracle Cushion

Stick Foundation

I like foundation sticks for several reasons: They usually have a creamy texture, they're ideal for spot coverage, and they're handy and portable—you can pop one in your makeup bag without fear that you'll later find a puddle of liquid foundation coating your lipstick and mascara.

A few **Best Bets:**

- Bobbi Brown Skin Foundation Stick
- Make Up For Ever Pan Stick Foundation
- Shiseido Stick Foundation
- Revlon PhotoReady Insta-Fix Makeup

Cream-to-Powder Foundation

A great cream-to-powder formula offers the best of both worlds: a glide-on start, and a nonshiny finish for those of us still experiencing oily skin. Apply with a sponge only where necessary or when going more golden. If you're covering the entire face, apply sparingly, but go heavier on the T-zone area (i.e., to even out redness on the cheeks or chin or to mitigate shine). Because they're housed in a compact, they're also portable and mess-free. One caveat: This formula is not for dry skin. Women with a drier complexion will want a more luminous finish and will be happier with one of the other formulas mentioned above, particularly a tinted moisturizer, liquid, or cream foundation.

Consider these **Best Bets:**

- Benefit Some Kind-A-Gorgeous the foundation faker
- CoverGirl CG Smoothers Aquasmooth Compact Foundation

- L'Oreal Paris True Match Super-Blendable Compact Makeup
- MAC Studio Fix Powder Plus Foundation

Brightening Foundation

These offer a radiance boost to the skin. Radiance, which is defined as fresh, luminous, glowing skin that looks youthful, is especially problematic for women over fifty, as the turnover rate of our skin cells has slowed and our skin has lost luminosity. However, be careful that the boost of radiance does not look fake or too shiny on your skin.

On my short list of **Best Bets:**

- CoverGirl + Olay Tone Rehab 2-in-1 Foundation
- Lancôme Teint Miracle Foundation
- Shiseido Future Solution LX Total Radiance Foundation SPF 20
- Giorgio Armani Luminous Silk Foundation
- Maybelline New York Instant Age Rewind Firming Makeup

Now that you've selected the type of foundation that meets your skincare needs, remember that less is definitely more when it comes to how much you use—especially after fifty. Let the fun begin!

mission accomplished . . . almost

To maximize the benefit of just having found the perfect cover for your skin, you should take advantage of a few easy steps to get more bang for your buck. Knowing how to ready your skin, how to choose an application tool or method, and how to assess your needs and make adjustments for even more perfect coverage can go the extra distance to the state of foundation bliss. Consider the following tips to add to your cosmetic skill set:

1 BE SURE TO EXFOLIATE

You are probably thinking, *What does exfoliating have to do with foundation?* A lot. By sloughing off dead skin cells once or twice a week, you are creating a smooth surface for your foundation to sit on. Makeup will go on evenly, and skin will look fresh, smooth, and glowing. But a word to the wise: Don't go heavy on the scrubs; stick with very mild exfoliants which don't irritate the skin like rice powders and InstantPeel (my favorite—and it comes in single-use packets). Or try the Clarisonic (www.clarisonic.com), a sonic cleansing brush that smoothes dead cells away. I use mine without soap or cleanser—just warm water. Heavy scrubs with abrasive ingredients can cause irritation and redness on the skin; anyone with dry skin should beware of those.

2 SELECT YOUR TOOL OF CHOICE

Fingers, sponge, or brush? It all depends on what type of foundation you're using and how much coverage you want. Be sure to consider the following before you choose which tool to use.

Fingertips:
Test used when applying liquid and cream foundations, because the heat from your fingertips warms up the pigment, making it easy to blend.

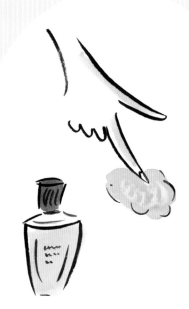

Sponge:

Best to achieve a sheer look, because it absorbs a lot of foundation. Lightly press it into the skin in a blotting/patting motion; don't sweep it across your face unless you want to create streaks. For a dewier look, dampen the sponge with water before dipping it into the foundation.

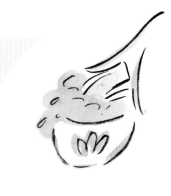

Brush:

Deposits the foundation most evenly and if you choose a tapered brush it allows you to expertly get around your nose and mouth area. "Paint" in light strokes on areas you need more coverage and then in sweeping motions, blend foundation into the skin until it's invisible.

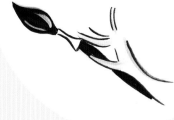

3 ASSESS AND TWEAK

Applying your foundation can be as simple as dabbing a dark spot here and there, or going full-frontal coverage to mask a bad skin day. Before applying your foundation, you need to assess what kind of coverage you think you need. There are bound to be days when you need more or less foundation coverage than usual.

Unless you live in a biosphere, or go around swathed from head to toe like a beekeeper, your complexion doesn't stay the same color year-round. So why should your foundation? It only makes sense that your makeup should shift in tone along with the seasons. When you're paler in the cool weather, you tone it down a shade. When the mercury rises, and your weekend hike has left you with a sun-kissed glow, you ratchet up the über flattering gold factor I discussed earlier.

You can also use a slight shade-tweak to help you fake it till you make it. For example, if you're chained to your desk all summer while all your friends are languishing at the beach, you can "cheat" by using a foundation a few shades darker than your everyday look. (This is why it's always important to buy one or two shades deeper than your standard color.) Nobody needs to know your beauty secrets but you.

Sometimes, your foundation needs will change overnight, literally: Perhaps a Sunday spent outdoors, sailing or skiing has left you a little windblown and ruddy, or maybe you had one too many cocktails at dinner last night and you need that extra face boost. Whether it's seasonal changes

Nobody needs to know your beauty secrets but you.

or day-to-day shifts in skin tone, don't be afraid to play "mixologist." You can blend a few drops of medium-coverage liquid foundation into your usual light-coverage tinted moisturizer, or even layer a bit of liquid over your crème-to-powder formula.

After applying your primer and concealer to cleansed and moisturized skin (as outlined in Chapter 4), start with a few dabs of foundation and build from there. Just make sure that when you first begin to experiment with mixing and applying your foundation, you do it in very bright natural light (a window or a skylight, for example). That way, when you step outside or anywhere else, you'll feel confident that your foundation is just the shade you want it to be. Before long, playing DIY makeup artist—and scaling up or down as necessary—will be second nature.

I HAVE TO admit, foundation is called foundation for a good reason—it is the baseline for all of your other beauty efforts, and it is *by far* the most important piece of the fifty+ beauty puzzle. Once you nail the right shades and formula, it's transformative in a way that no other product can touch—like a blissful vacation or the morning after. By showing the world the aspects of your face that you really love, and keeping all that other stuff lightly under wraps, you are taking a huge, vibrant, confident leap forward for your face.

Now that you've found the perfect white T-shirt of your beauty routine, read on for beauty tips for eyes, lips, and cheeks. After all, a perfect white T-shirt is great on its own, but paired with a J Crew jacket, it's unstoppable.

A WORD ON ANTIAGING TREATMENT FOUNDATION

"Treatment" foundations are the darling du jour of the cosmetics companies. A mash-up of skin care and makeup, treatment foundations are often laced with the same high-tech ingredients found in pricey antiaging elixirs. On paper, they sound fabulous—what time-starved woman doesn't want to try to kill two beauty birds with one stone? But while this all sounds great, antiaging treatment foundations don't usually deliver. Simply put, no foundation can lift, firm, or eliminate your lines and wrinkles—period.

A word of caution: Once you start layering treatment foundations on top of the skin care you're already using, you could be setting yourself up for irritation. (Case in point: Retinol, which is frequently included in treatment foundations, should really only be used at night because it renders the skin photosensitive.)

Having said all that, I'm not completely down on treatment foundations. In fact, there are two skincare ingredients that I absolutely swear by in makeup: SPF and hyaluronic acid. Of course you know why you need the former—to short-circuit the formation of additional lines and wrinkles, while hyaluronic acid is a world-class skin plumper and a total moisture magnet. Plump, moist, and sun-protected equals gorgeous fifty+ skin.

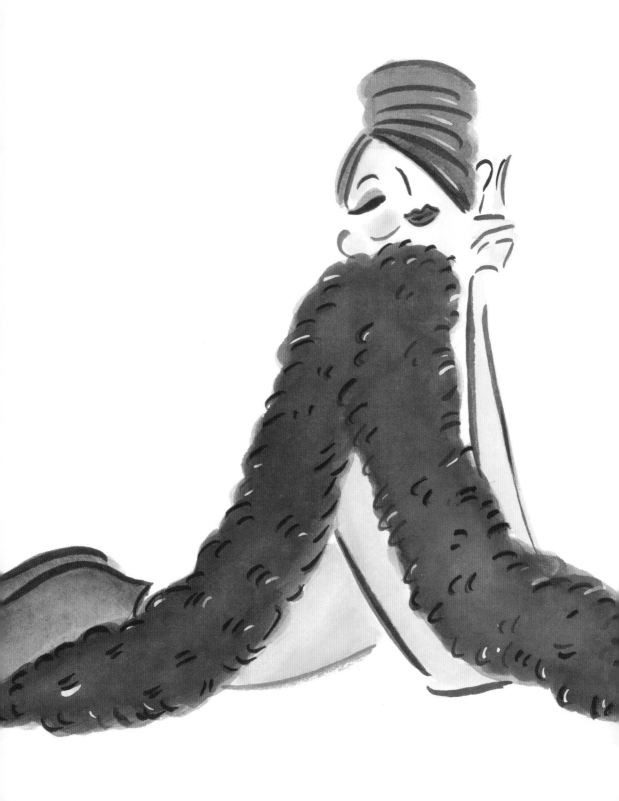

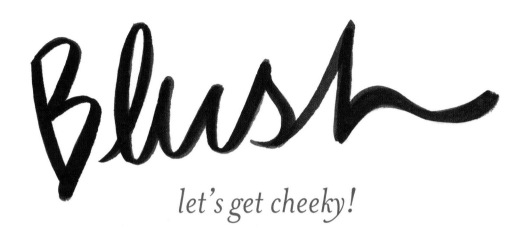

CHAPTER SIX

Blush

let's get cheeky!

YOUR CHEEKS, UNLIKE YOUR ASS, SHOULD ALWAYS BE PLUMP! PLUMP, FRESH, AND GORGEOUS.

But the cheeks you were born with aren't the same cheeks you see in the mirror once you're over fifty, and, like a host of other body parts, they tend to move south as your birthdays move north.

Like squeezing into a flattering pair of J Brand jeans, knowing how to add the right color and texture where it counts can give the illusion of great "cheeks" and accentuate your assets. Great looking cheeks, both

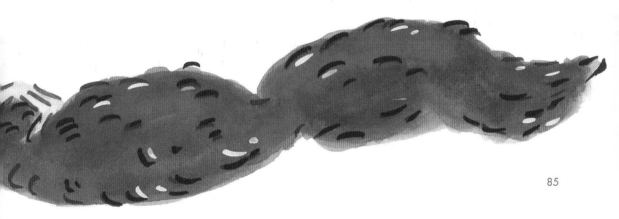

upper and lower, equal good, healthy sex appeal. This chapter will tell you everything you need to know about how to find the right cheek color, how to layer color and use texture, how to highlight, and how to choose the cheek products that will make your face glow because that's exactly what you want now—believable glow, radiance, and luminosity—that "just ran a couple of miles" look.

So, cheeky is a good thing—it really is. Bringing out your cheeks is an easy and essential step for looking your absolute best at fifty+. If you've never worn blush before, you *must* start working it into your daily beauty routine. To me, blush, like taxes, jury duty, and making it to your Pilates class, is *not* optional.

Okay, I'm prejudiced. Blush has always been the cosmetic placeholder of my youth. Perhaps it's my seven-year-old self's memory of my mother with her tiny round cardboard box of what she called "rouge," and her deliberate swirls of the little cotton pad on her face, transforming her beauty. Perhaps it's Julie Christie's cheeks in *Dr. Zhivago.* Perhaps it's because I remember my first kiss on my cheek from Michael Egan when I was twelve.

But even if all my makeup memories didn't somehow circle back to blush, I'd still think it was of primary importance in the grand hierarchy of cosmetics. Because from my experience, there is no other single piece of makeup that is more useful in creating the illusion of youth than blush, when well applied. It is the take-your-breath-away beauty element in your makeup regimen. It is your face's softness, innocence, vulnerability, and natural beauty. For these reasons, using blush and choosing the right color is the face-defining factor—really you, only better. Blush is entirely underrated but incredibly important, so make a mantra of the following . . .

BEAUTY TRUTH:

Getting cheeky is essential to capturing the youth quotient.

For most of us, that is . . . but here's one for the books that gives new meaning to "getting cheeky." This is a true story that happened to a friend (and executive) in the cosmetics industry.

She once had to supervise a campaign shoot for cheek color—a new launch that the company she was working for was sinking a lot of money into with the belief that a certain celebrity spokesperson (who shall remain nameless) with a huge contract (hundreds of thousands, for ten days of work) would do a good job of selling to the public (us). But when it came time to shoot the commercial, the starlet refused to say the name of the product! She even threatened to walk off the set, despite the fact that her dressing room had been stocked with Cristal champagne and Petrossian Caviar at her request. When she finally was convinced to come on set after a heated exchange between the company's legal counsel and her agent, she wanted to keep all the clothes—even the one-of-a-kind original samples we had borrowed from designers. And when the stylist sent her a bill for the shoes and clothing, she promptly handed it over to us and threatened to skip out on the remaining days of her contract if we didn't pay for her shopping spree! She was not the sweet "blushing" girl we all had read about in *People* magazine. No, I will not reveal the identity of this self-absorbed diva, but let's face it—there is cheeky and then there is CHEEKY!

Unlike getting this starlet to cooperate, blush, by contrast, requires very little fuss to get it to deliver. It's an easy-breezy do, and the quickest to apply of all the cosmetic products—just dab, blend, and possibly highlight. Forget trying to contour or sculpt;

it will never look good. Avoid being that woman with the two streaks of color on her face. Run away from this look fast and leave it to celebrity makeup artists. You are not posing for a magazine; you are a real woman living your life!

What *is* critical is choosing your texture and color. Since those buoyant, plump, round cheeks of yore are starting to move downward, we are going to rely on our cosmetic wits to master and restore this lovable part of the face.

the art of blushing

Want to look really old? Use powder blush. Your skin is likely not as smooth as it once was, and perhaps has a few lines and rough patches as well. Powder blush will sit in those lines, and your cheeks will end up looking splotchy and uneven. Never use powder blush again. Go into your makeup closet right this minute and toss that powder blush. Replace it with creams, sticks, and tints—that's all you need. They are mistake-proof, and starting with a little controllable dab, you can easily build to a visible natural color.

Read on for the highlights of how to select and apply blush for best effect.

1 IDENTIFY YOUR COLOR PALETTE

Here are a few color tips that will help you hone in on the right hue for your skin tone:

If you have FAIR skin:

- DO start by trying out dusty pink shades or woody rose tones.
- DON'T choose shades that are ruby or purple in hue, as these shades only create a bruised appearance on the skin.

If you have MEDIUM skin:

- DO go for tawnier tones similar to the yellow undertones in your skin, like apricot, clay, and burnt coral colors.
- DON'T use dark shades, pastels, and very light pinks, which offset the warmth in your skin color.

If you have DARK skin:

- DO try more deep and intense shades, like bronze and golden shades; deep plums, burgundies, and ruby reds work well, too.
- DON'T use pastels and bright pinks, as these shades may create a washed out or chalky appearance on your skin.

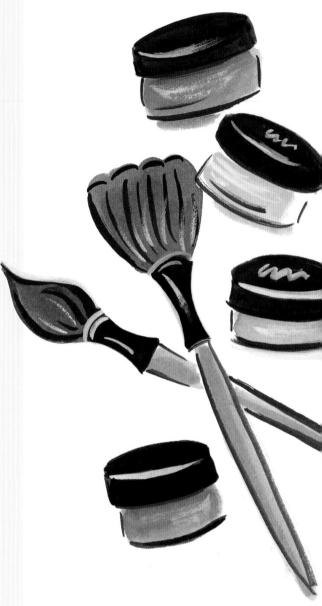

I admit I am a sucker for a neutral palette even on the darkest skin, so make sure the intense colors also have a neutral cast to them. Often, women with darker skin tones feel compelled to use bright colors. Rethink this. There is nothing prettier than a dot of healthy neutral color (in deeper intensities) on the cheeks of very dark skin. Try a burgundy to the brown side; you may be very surprised—the more neutral, the more natural.

Another good tip for choosing a cheek color: If you have a favorite tried-and-true lip color, pick a blush in the same family. This creates more harmony on the face. Also, try to pick up colors that will look good with your hair. For example, redheads should stick with the colors of highlights in their hair (rosy and/or peachy).

Now that you have an idea of your correct color palette, it's time to determine what type of blush consistency will best suit your skin type.

2 SELECT A TEXTURE

Assuming you've all tossed out your powder blushes like I recommended above (Not yet? I'll wait. Done? Okay), it's time to choose a consistency and type of blush that works best for your skin and lifestyle. As I mentioned, both creams and sticks work much the same way, so it's really just finding what type of application form you prefer. Some find sticks easier to use and quicker to apply, while others enjoy the flexibility of creams, since they're easier to mix with foundation or moisturizer. It's up to you.

Cream Blushes:

These products come in a variety of consistencies, from very shiny to more matte creams, so it is a question of finding which works best with your skin type. For example, super dry skin should not use the matte textures because this consistency, like powder blush, will sit in your lines and not move over dry patches. Creams also do not last as long as powder, so know that you may have to retouch a few times a day to hold the intensity. And one more thing you should know is that you can't always count on the color in the pot being the color you get on your face, so trying it before you buy it is imperative. If you can't try it before purchasing and feel you've made a mistake, return it or try this: If it is too intense, blend foundation into the color; if too pale, mix it with darker lipstick.

Here are a few **Best Bets** in cream-based blush products:
- Laura Mercier Crème Cheek Colour (my favorite shade is Praline)
- MAC Cremeblend Blush in Ladyblush
- Maybelline New York Dream Bouncy Blush
- Revlon Cream Blush

Stick Blushes:

This form of blush is similar to a cream blush and most often less oily in consistency; like lipstick, it also comes in a container that is portable, and it aids in controlling the "messy" factor during application. It is a bit dryer in texture than cream, and one quick dab on each cheek usually distributes enough color that can be quickly blended with the fingers. Like creams, sticks come in a variety of finishes that require some trial and error to see what works best for your skin. A word of caution: Avoid the sticks that have a high level of shimmer.

On my short list of good stick blushes:
- Clinique Blushwear Cream Stick
- NARS The Multiple
- NYX Stick Blush

3 FIND YOUR SWEET SPOT AND APPLY

Look in the mirror and smile—just trust me. Now put your
finger on the apple, or "sweet spot," of your cheek.
It's located just a hair under your cheekbone (the apple
might have to move a little higher as time passes). Rub
your fingers in a circular motion on that spot until you
see a small blush of color begin to develop and notice
where it is most intense. This is the "sweet spot" where
you'll dab a small amount of your blush and blend it.
With creams and sticks, your best application tool is your
clean finger or a washable flat silk sponge, and the objective is
to blend your cheek color seamlessly into your moisturized face
(or into your foundation or tinted moisturizer), so the blush is natural
looking and has soft edges. (Note that creamy formulas can warm to a more intense hue with
the heat of our body, so apply sparingly and build the color gradually and carefully.) Dab the
cream blush on with your middle finger and then blend with your pointer, middle, and ring
fingers. Use a circular motion, building color, and feathering the edges for softness. This is the
key to beautiful, natural-looking cheeks. Easy, right? Read on for further tips and tricks to maximize your cheekiness.

Experiment with glow by taking a small swipe of your natural, low-shimmer highlighter (or
another very shiny cream blush) and move it in a circular motion across the cheekbone for an
extra shot of youthfulness. This attracts light the way young luminous skin does. (I use Laura
Mercier Crème Cheek Colour and then use another more shiny cheek color, MAC Cremeblend
Blush, as my highlighter). If you want a healthy, sun-kissed look, apply your blush, and then
swipe bronzer lightly on top of your cheek color. You can also try the reverse—bronzer first with
cream blush on top. Which way looks best? It depends on you and your blush. Another trick,
one I favor, is to catch your foundation or tinted moisturizer before it has completely dried and
mix the blush right into it, forming a completely natural look. In other words, it is the immediate
next step after applying your foundation.

THE TINIEST CHANGE can often make a huge difference, and this is the way I feel about blush. Just moving from powder to cream moves your look forward and into the more natural sphere. You'll also find that it takes less time, and I am a great believer in our hand getting in touch with the planes of our face. That's how we get to know it and love it.

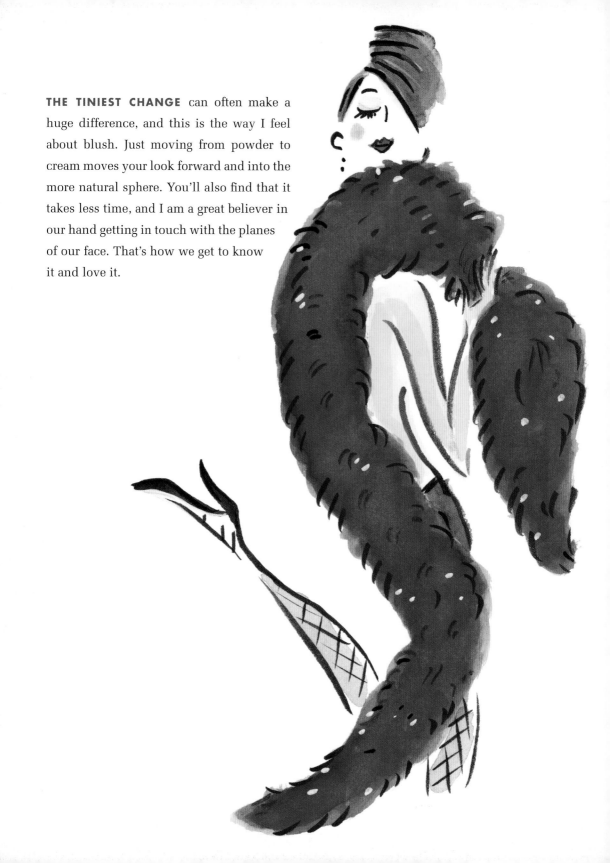

YOU SHOULD KNOW

When it comes to shopping for blush products, here's a beauty truth worth knowing about: Cosmetic companies annually (sometimes twice a year) do "category reviews" on best-selling shades among their competitors and then incorporate those bestsellers into their product lineup. The catch? These luxury brands now view drugstore brands as competitors since consumers increasingly shop for cosmetics at both high-end department stores like Saks as well as drugstores like CVS, so you are likely to find the same bestselling cheek shades from brands like Maybelline and L'Oreal as you might from a higher-end manufacturer, like Lancôme.

Additionally, did you know that many companies don't produce or create their own powder cheek colors? They go to a handful of vendors (mostly Italian) with expertise in finely milled powders to source them. The end product you see—whether it's $10 or $75, whether it's headed to CVS or Saks—likely came from the same supplier/factory with many of the same formulas and colors.

Talk about being cheeky!

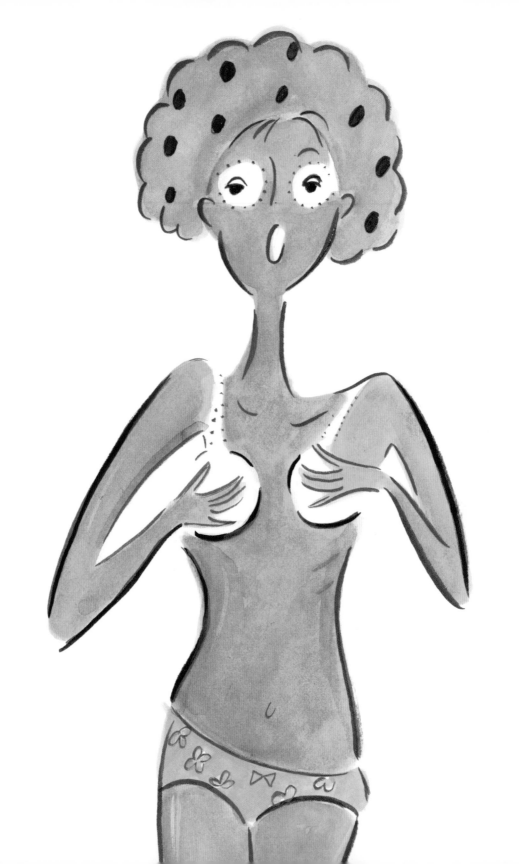

CHAPTER SEVEN

TANNING

the ultimate fake bake

WANT TO KNOW THE MOST GLAMOROUS WAY TO GET SKIN CANCER? LAY OUT ON A YACHT DECK IN SAINT TROPEZ, SLATHERED IN BABY OIL AND IODINE.

Okay, it's a bit dramatic, and frankly, I shouldn't even have to say it—by now you should know: Don't sit in the sun unprotected. Never, never, never!

Tanning is no longer an option unless you want crocodile skin. Though you may find it appealing on a pair of Jimmy Choo boots, you definitely don't want to see scaley skin on your face, so one more time: No tanning! Not on the beach, not in a tanning bed, not anywhere—not allowed. But you are allowed to still have a gorgeous, sun-kissed glow that adds an exotic aura and sensuality to your skin. It's no secret that a good "tan" can hide a multitude of sins, including yellow teeth, uneven skin tone, red spots, and veins. And with a great healthy glow, you don't need to wear foundation, which is a luxury in itself. (It will also make your eye color look more intense.)

A little bronzer is the quickest and easiest way to give your skin a bit of golden color.

This chapter discusses how to achieve that fabulous fake bake using a variety of products without damaging your skin. Of course, that sunny radiance isn't easy to achieve, so you have to start a relationship with one or perhaps all of the following backups: a good bronzer, a great self-tanner, and a golden-tinted moisturizer.

I will teach you how to layer these products to customize just the right tone for your skin so that you can achieve a year-round golden glow. For instance, did you know that you can layer a self-tanner with an illuminating bronzer for even more glow? And, since it goes without saying that you still need to wear sunscreen every day, I'll give you that list, too. But first, let's start with the obvious: bronzer.

bronzers

A little bronzer is the quickest and easiest way to give your skin a bit of golden color. Remember, golden is the path to radiance and youth, but be careful. Going too orange or too red with your bronzer can make you look like an Oompa Loompa, so avoid this pitfall. The trick is choosing the right golden hue for your skin tone and applying it properly. If you are fair, select a bronzer that has rosy-gold or peach undertones. If you have medium skin, use a bronze or copper shade, and, with dark skin, go for a bronzer that has deep rust and deep copper undertones. Steer clear of sparkle, glitter, and high shimmer—that's for high school.

a great healthy glow . . .

CREAM BRONZERS

These will give you a glow that you won't get from powder, and they are especially great for dry skin, which most of us have after age fifty. This consistency may come in a stick as well as a pot. Apply it on the areas of the face and décolletage where the sun would naturally fall. Blend it on the cheek bones, lightly on the temples, and sweep it across the bridge of your nose—but only if it has a low-level or no shimmer. Most bronzers do have some shimmer pigment, so if you choose one with shimmer, skip the bridge of your nose. I love the look of bronzer mixed with blush—try mixing the two (cream with cream) for a subtle, healthy flush. Best application tools are fingertips and/or a sponge.

Best Bets:

- NARS The Multiple in Na Pali Coast, South Beach, and Portofino
- Sonia Kashuk Undetectable Crème Bronzer

LIQUID BRONZERS

These come as gels, tints, and serums and are usually the sheerest formulas, great for everyday wear. Gels (which also come in stick form) are best suited for oilier skin types, which few of us are at this stage of life. They are packaged in a tube or bottle and often look darker than the color that you want, but they are often more translucent and lighter than they appear, and give your skin the sheerest wash of color. Try mixing your foundation or tinted moisturizer with a liquid bronzer, but again make sure the bronzer has little to no shimmer if you are going to use it all over your face. Start with a small amount and build from there. Here, too, sponge and fingertips work equally well for application.

A few **Best Bets:**

- Dr. Hauschka Translucent Bronzing Tint
- Giorgio Armani Fluid Sheer 10 (good for medium to dark skin tones)
- Givenchy Mister Radiant (good for light skin tones)
- Laura Mercier Bronzing Gel

POWDER BRONZERS

As you've probably gathered, I am not a fan of powder for cheeks, face, or for bronzing, and, unfortunately, powder bronzer is probably the most common form found in department stores and drugstores. Those big compacts that won't fit in a purse have enough product to last red-carpet starlets Snooki and JWoww combined for the next decade. Plus, powder on top of dry skin will make you look old and cannot be easily blended. Most often it looks really fake. So if you cannot find a bronzer that's anything but powder, go for a finely milled dewy bronzing powder that will blend seamlessly with your tinted moisturizer or foundation, once they have dried after application, and try lightly dusting it over your blush for just a hint of a healthy glow. Use a big fluffy brush and tap off any excess product before using. Concentrate the color at your temples and along your cheekbones. And without double dipping, lightly brush across your nose and chin. As always, do not choose a powder with detectable shimmer or glitter!

Choose among these **Best Bets:**

- Benefit Hoola Bronzing Powder
- Bobbi Brown Bronzing Powder
- Guerlain Terracotta Bronzing Powder
- NARS Bronzing Powder in Laguna
- Tom Ford Bronzing Powder in Terra
- Physician's Formula Cashmere Wear Ultra-Smoothing Bronzer

Whatever bronzer you choose to go with, the key to getting that perfect faux glow is not just about having the right product, it's also knowing how to apply it well and use it properly. Here are a few tips to achieving the right amount of radiance:

do not choose a powder with detectable shimmer or glitter . . .

1 A bronzer should be used to look healthier, not tanner.

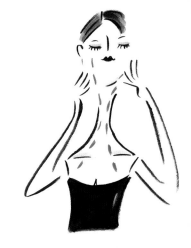

2 Avoid ending up with a different colored face and neck by extending your bronzing strokes lightly down the face to the neck and on to the collarbone.

3 Apply your bronzer lightly, building up your color slowly; it's easier to add color than it is to take it away.

4 Skip bronzer altogether if you have any skin eruptions, large pores, or your skin is misbehaving.

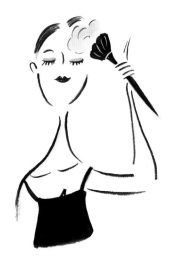

5 If you can't find a shade of bronzer that looks perfectly natural on your skin, try mixing two colors of the same consistency.

6 For a more subtle glow, mix liquid bronzer with your moisturizer or your primer, and then follow with foundation or tinted moisturizer.

7 For a more intense glow, skip the primer and try mixing liquid bronzer with your foundation or tinted moisturizer.

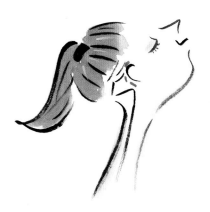

8 If your hair will be styled in a ponytail, twist, or knot, use bronzer on the ears and the back of the neck.

9 Always apply bronzer in natural light.

self-tanners

Here's a confession: I had gotten the message early about the damaging effects of sunbathing and tanning beds, so I became a spray-tan addict—along with Lindsay Lohan and every other reality TV star and red carpet disaster. I was hooked—I mean *really* hooked. At least once a week, I would step into a booth, strip down to nothing, extend my arms out like a scarecrow, and hold my breath as the tanning spray misted me from head to toe. Then I'd turn around and do it on the other side. I felt like one of those rotisserie chickens at Whole Foods.

And much like dessert portions, the method for finding the line where a little becomes too much is the key to success.

But then one day, I discovered something unsettling that made me go cold turkey (or cold chicken, in this case). Sure, I'd been willing to suffer through the embalming solution smell for the first six hours and had put up with it when the tanning solution stained my Egyptian cotton sheets orange, along with my ankles and heels. I was undaunted! Unstoppable! Even after my blond highlights went umber in that mist, ruining Louis Licari's sophisticated handiwork on my hair. What ultimately undid me, after a year of addiction, was being handed a pair of nose clips to wear when I checked in at the salon for my weekly spray down. With this little gesture, my beauty routine was transformed into a HazMat situation. I panicked! What exactly was I breathing in? Were Lindsay and I going to be victims of "orange lung" disease—or worse?

Once I discovered the deleterious side effects of indulging in spray tans (beyond orange heels and ruined sheets, I was inhaling possible cancer-causing chemicals), I quit and moved to at-home DIY self-tanning. Better to have "orange hand" than "orange lung."

Despite all this drama, nothing beats a little healthy glow on the body and face at this stage of life. The operative point here is "a little." And much like dessert portions, the method for finding the line where a little becomes too much is the key to success.

The best way to navigate this category without looking like a pumpkin is by using tanning lotions that provide *gradual* color, and by applying them properly. Here are some take-home tanning tips that will help you avoid the orange menace:

TEST

If this is your first adventure into the world of sunless tanning, test the product on a hidden spot on your body to be sure the color and shade is right for you and that you have no allergic reaction.

EXFOLIATE

This is often overlooked and it is a very important step. By exfoliating in the days before applying a self-tanner, you will ensure your tan looks even and lasts longer. When you rub away dead skin cells, the new layer of skin will absorb the formula more efficiently.

MOISTURIZE

After each exfoliation you need to hydrate the skin to expedite the absorption of the formula and to leave skin looking ultra smooth and glowing.

WASH HANDS

To avoid orange stains or streaks, wash your hands every five minutes when applying the self-tanner, and don't forget the area between the fingers, fingernails, cuticles and knuckles. Or use surgical gloves. Personally, I find it difficult to apply lotion with gloves, but many have mastered this.

BEWARE OF BENDABLE AREAS

Go easy when spreading the self-tanning formula around your knees, armpits, ankles, feet, and elbows, as the thicker the skin, the more it absorbs the color, which then leaves you with dark-orange areas. You can also apply a light layer of lotion to these areas beforehand to help dilute the product.

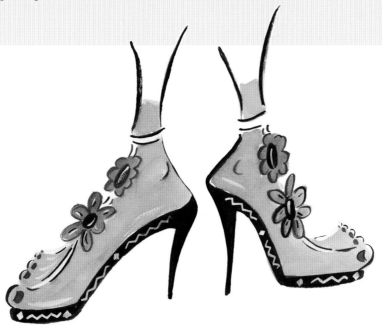

Now that you know the best practices of self-tanning application, you'll need to choose among the dizzying array of products out there and decide whether you want instant gratification or a slow-to-grow glow. All come with manageable pros and cons, and most brands offer a standard skin color range: fair, medium, or dark.

GRADUAL SELF-TANNING LOTIONS

As mentioned earlier, the key to good color, in my opinion, is to build the glow slowly with daily use. Like any beauty venture, there are pros and cons to different methods. With gradual color, the advantage is that you'll see minimal streaking, blotchiness, and buildup on ankles, souls of the feet, and knuckles. The downside? Patience. You're going to have to be patient—it takes a few days to arrive at the color you want, and you must reapply the self-tanner every day. The good news: These products are made to moisturize, so you can cut the moisturizing step out of your daily beauty routine. Also, they often contain a sunscreen, so you can eliminate this step as well. This category is very affordable, almost foolproof, and can be found easily at your local CVS, Duane Reade, or Walgreens.

Consider these **Best Bets:**
- L'Oreal Sublime Bronze Tinted Self-Tanning Lotion
- Coppertone Gradual Tan Moisturizing Lotion
- Jergens Natural Glow Daily Moisturizing Lotion

In my opinion, *gradual* self-tanning is the way to go. BUT, if for some reason you jump immediately to an instant self-tanner, I would exercise extreme moderation until you have found a color and method of application that's right for you. I am not trying to be a killjoy, but these products can get us into trouble. And by trouble, I mean Oompa Loompa orange: dark-orange elbows, orange knuckles, orange knees, orange ankles, and even face, if you apply too liberally. Guard against getting it in your eyebrows, as well, as blond eyebrows will turn orange. Also, instant self-tanners are not so instant; they usually take several hours to activate to full color and will last several days (a week)

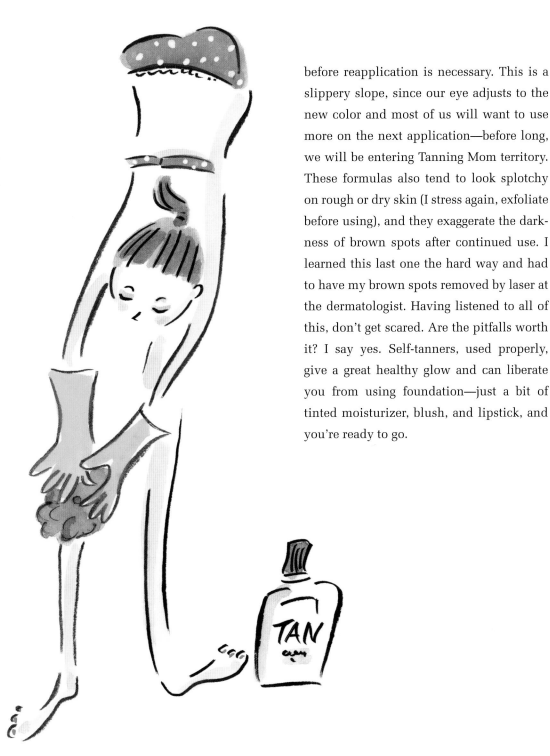

before reapplication is necessary. This is a slippery slope, since our eye adjusts to the new color and most of us will want to use more on the next application—before long, we will be entering Tanning Mom territory. These formulas also tend to look splotchy on rough or dry skin (I stress again, exfoliate before using), and they exaggerate the darkness of brown spots after continued use. I learned this last one the hard way and had to have my brown spots removed by laser at the dermatologist. Having listened to all of this, don't get scared. Are the pitfalls worth it? I say yes. Self-tanners, used properly, give a great healthy glow and can liberate you from using foundation—just a bit of tinted moisturizer, blush, and lipstick, and you're ready to go.

INSTANT SELF-TANNERS

Within the world of instant self-tanners, there is a wide range of choices and forms available—lotions, creams, liquids, gels, mousses (foams), aerosol spray tans, and tan towels. Your selection should be based on the easiest application method for you to handle, your natural skin color, and the hoped-for result, which should be an even, healthy glow. Like the gradual tanning lotions (which by far are my first choice), they most often come with a skin-color code. You never want to go more than a couple of shades darker than your natural skin color—more than that begins to look fake.

Self-Tanning Towelettes

I personally prefer the tan towels, since they can be used easily with surgical gloves (no orange palms), and their solution spreads evenly and dries quickly. They come in packets for different parts of the body (face, arms, or legs), which is a great benefit for travel. When using the towel, be sure to reach into corners of the face and cover the surface of the ears. Use very carefully around the hairline and around the neck and décolletage. The downside of the tan towel is that it is drying, so it's wise to use a liberal dose of moisturizer once the color has reached its full potential.

Best Bets:

- Dr. Dennis Gross Skincare Alpha Beta Glow Pad
- Kate Somerville 360° Face Self Tanning Pads

Lotions and Creams

These products are convenient, and, if you have really dry skin, they're better than using self-tanning towelettes because they bring instant moisture to the equation. The downside? The chances of streaking, uneven color, and blotching are greater because, as you rub the product in, it's hard to know what areas you have already covered until it begins to show up. So you'll need to establish a routine for your application, working your way either up your body or down. As you become more adept at your application, this routine will become habit, and you'll find that you miss fewer spots and provide more even coverage over your skin. Be aware—that like spray tanning, these self-tanning products can stain your clothes, towels, and bed sheets, so be sure to let the product dry before getting dressed or going to bed.

Best Bets worth considering:

- Jergens Natural Glow FACE Daily Facial Moisturizing with SPF 20
- Jergens Natural Glow Daily Moisturizing Lotion
- Nivea Sun-Kissed Radiance Gradual Tanner and Body Lotion

Gels and Mousses

People with oily or eruption-prone menopausal skin usually prefer a gel or mousse (or tan towel) because they usually contain less oil, making them less likely to clog pores. An added benefit— they spread and dry quickly. These forms offer the same coverage power of lotions or creams without the downside of too many humectants.

Here are a few of my favorites:

- Clarins Self Tanning Instant Gel
- L'Oreal Sublime Bronze Clear Self-Tanning Gel
- St. Tropez Bronzing Mousse
- Clinique Face Bronzing Gel

Aerosols

Personally, spray tans in an aerosol remind me too much of the tanning booth. I don't like breathing in the mist, the notion of ruining the ozone layer, or doing damage to the walls of my bathroom and shower, which will take on a vague orange color like the pollution haze at sunset in Los Angeles. Be forewarned about this. That said, they . . . enough said.

HOW LONG DOES a faux tan last with any one of the above choices? Five to seven days. Reapplying before that (other than touching up missed spots) will start you on that very slippery downhill slope that tripped up Lindsay and me.

So proceed with caution and learn how to master the fine art of tanning without the fears that accompany harmful ultra violet rays of the sun. Of course, it goes without saying that you *must* still wear sunscreen every day. It's like a credit card or a fully charged cell phone—you don't want to leave home without it. Used wisely, self-tanners are a great tool for the warm weather months and a healthy pick-me-up for changing skin tone and color. And yes, if you *really* are daunted by the self-tanning trial and error, simply stick to your tinted moisturizer or foundation in a golden shade. But I didn't dedicate an entire chapter of this book because I wanted to skip my grueling Pilates workout—I did it because I know it's one of the best things you can do to look more vibrant, sexy, vigorous, and youthful. The bottom line? A great self-tan can do wonders for your confidence. But much like cheesecake and chocolate mousse, it's best to indulge in it with moderation.

a great self-tan can do wonders for your confidence . . . .

Odor alert! The chemical agent (DHA) that triggers the tanning action of many self-tanners has a distinct and pungent smell similar to that of hair color chemicals in salons, but in my darkest thoughts I imagine it smells a little like embalming fluid. Then again, I have no idea what that smells like. This smell takes several showers to eliminate, so be prepared to camouflage that odor with your favorite fragrance—or avoid mingling in close quarters with others until it dissipates. Some products, however, boast mild to no smell. If after-scent is an issue to you, be sure to test it with your own nose before purchasing.

Sometimes, self-tanning goes wrong: streaks, blotchiness, and dark-orange smudges on the ankles, heels, and between the fingers, to name a few. Don't hide behind gloves, socks, or a muumuu if this happens to you! There *are* remedies. While the newest self-tanning formulas are easier to apply and somewhat foolproof, mistakes do happen. Should this happen to you, here are a few tips for dialing down the damage:

- Rub lemon juice, rubbing alcohol, or an alpha hydroxy acid cream over the area to minimize the smudging and/or streaking.

- Exfoliate and try to get the pigments out by sloughing off skin cells. Whether you use a loofah, body scrub, or plain old baking soda on a washcloth, this action will allow newer (untanned) skin cells to surface more rapidly.

- Use a self-tan remover. Several companies offer tan remover pads or creams to help lift the pigment away from the skin. Try Tanwise Tan Remover from Sally Beauty for your palms or Uh Oh Self Tan Remover.

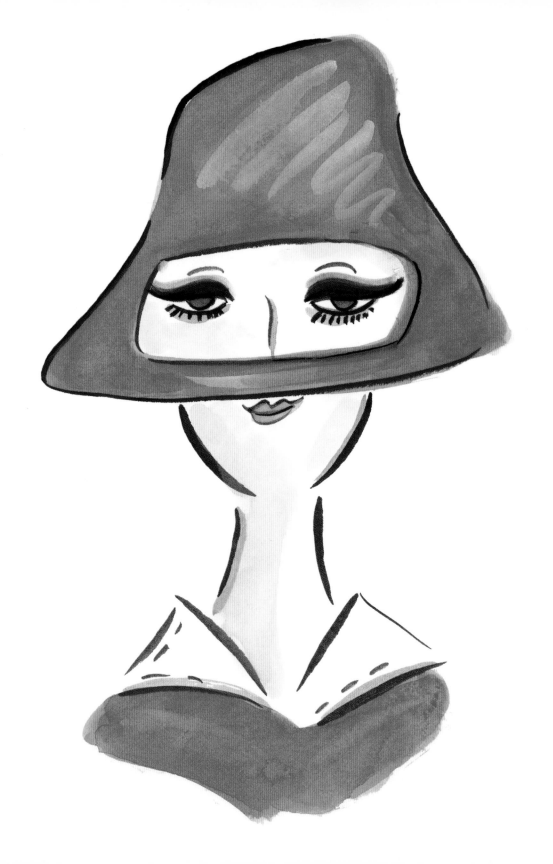

CHAPTER EIGHT

The Eyes Have It

eyeliner, eye shadow, mascara

A FEW YEARS AGO, I OBSERVED A "WOMAN OF A CERTAIN AGE" SURROUNDED BY THE MOST ATTRACTIVE MEN IN THE ROOM, ALL OF WHOM SEEMED OBVIOUSLY CHARMED BY HER.

It was at a cocktail party given by my boss and his wife, whom I was staying with for the weekend. There were plenty of "pretty young things" at the party (emphasis on the "young"), so I wondered what made her so alluring. I later found out from the hostess that she'd already had five husbands! (I wish I could tell you who this very social Mrs. X was, but revealing her name would put me in the witness protection program.) Having recently come out of a divorce myself, from a husband of many years, you can imagine my curiosity. As it turned out, she was staying the weekend as well, and, being fresh on the dating scene, I took the occasion to ask her for some advice. Here's what she told me: "It's all about the eyes. When I see someone attractive across the room, I stare

"I may not always have the right shoes, but I always have the right mascara."

until they notice me. When they do, I smile, and most often they follow." And wow oh wow did she work those eyes! She said, "I may not always have the right shoes, but I always have the right mascara."

For many of us, when we look in the mirror, our eyes do the opposite of wooing—they trigger a litany of complaints instead: bags, crow's feet, crêpe-y lids, and wimpy lashes. Here's where you want to take a deep breath, inhale, exhale, and listen: Eyes should be celebrated, not disparaged, so let's embrace this thought and learn how to love the eyes that we have.

In this chapter, I'll teach you simple, eye-opening makeup tips to help you accentuate the most expressive part of your face. It will include the products, the tools, and the application instruction you need to turn your eyes from tired to glamorous. If eyes can provoke battles, inspire songs, seduce lovers, and be the windows to the soul, don't you think it's worth the effort? Mrs. X got this concept in spades.

That said, Mrs. X wasn't *completely* candid with me on the mascara thing, as I found out later when I asked to borrow a hairdryer from the closet in her bathroom. She made the mistake of leaving her cosmetics bag out on the counter, and of course I locked the bathroom door and determined very quickly she wasn't just wearing mascara. Most of the products in her cosmetics case were indeed eye makeup, but she did such a great job using it that all you noticed were her gorgeous eyes and not her makeup. This is what I discovered in Mrs. X's makeup bag:

it's all about the eyes . . . .

- A duo eye-shadow palette in a neutral pair of light and medium tones (flesh and medium brown)

- A single shadow in a deep brown

- Three brushes: a shadow brush, a very thin liner brush, and an angled brush

- Lid primer

- Concealer

- Mascara

- Brow gel

- Eyelash curler

- Eyelash comb

Quite a lineup for our natural-looking, mascara-wearing Mrs. X, wasn't it? As the weekend progressed, I felt comfortable enough to ask her what she did with her eyes, besides flirting. She offered to share her tricks (about eye makeup, that is) and here's what I learned: She stated at the outset that the overarching goal was to use eye makeup in an upward and outward motion so the eyes looked bright, youthful, and open. I registered this as a very important clue since I had already noticed that it wasn't in my best interest to follow the downward direction of my upper eyelids. Here's Mrs. X's routine in more detail:

1 She reached for the primer first and applied it lightly to the lid all the way up to the brow to smooth and camouflage the fine lines. She gently patted it in with her ring finger.

2 This was followed by mixing the duo colors together with the shadow brush and applying the blended shades to the upper lid, up to the crease. This gave a very soft and pretty definition to the eye.

3 She then took the angled brush, dipped it into the dark single shadow, and applied a thin line along the upper lash line.

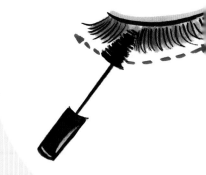

4 When she reached the outer corner of the eye, she blended in a bit more of the dark shadow and "winged" it out in a barely visible stroke. The goal of this, she mentioned, is to give the illusion of "lifting" the eye up, but not true cat eyes effect. (Leave that to your daughter along with liquid eyeliner.)

5 She then dipped the thin brush into the dark single eye shadow and lightly lined the lower lashes from the outer edges to three-quarters of the way to the inner corner of the eye, making the soft line thinner as it moved toward the inner corner.

6 Before using mascara, she curled her lashes. Her mascara routine was unlike any I had seen before—she applied the wand close to the lash line and moved it back and forth several times before pulling it through the lashes and followed up by holding the wand vertically and moving it back and forth like a windshield wiper (she claimed this rid the lashes of excess mascara and ensured that the tips were coated).

7 Next, Mrs. X applied a dot of concealer on the outer edges of her eyes, just under the uplifted shadow to emphasize the upward direction of her eyes.

8 She then added a dot of concealer on the inner corner next to the nose and blended it well to remove any darkness there (she emphasized that this step makes the eyes stand out).

9 Mrs. X finished her routine with a tiny bit of brow gel, which she used to gently sculpt her brows in—yes, that's right—an upward and outward direction, just like her shadow routine.

I can't say this routine will get you five more husbands (and really, who wants THAT), but I can say it's the easiest and most foolproof route to beautiful eye makeup. I've passed this lesson on to several grateful friends and colleagues, including makeup artists. Mrs. X was not a makeup artist, not a model, not a magazine editor, nor a beauty company executive. She was a woman of a certain age who had taught herself to master the art of eye makeup. The makeup was brilliant because it made you notice HER: her expression (happy and youthful), her beautiful eye color (green), and her pretty lashes. You didn't notice her crêpe-y eyelids or her crow's feet, which were there but camouflaged with the few strategic steps I've just outlined. But the most important piece of information I can share is that none of the steps had to be precise. The shadows she selected were so subtle (flesh and browns) that they blended seamlessly on to the lids, and a little bit of smudging did not harm the overall effect, which made for the most perfectly imperfect *Wabi-Sabi* eyes.

This is the method I have used every day (well . . . almost every day) since my encounter with Mrs. X, who luckily still remains married to her most recent happy husband.

Here are a few additional tips I picked up along the way as a beauty editor:

TO MAKE SMALL EYES BIGGER:

After primer, use the flesh or light gray part of your duo to cover the upper lid. Use the darker brown or dark gray/black to line the crease of the upper eye lid (A). Next, shade the outer corner of the lid and the crease with the darker brown or dark gray/black and blend well (B). Use the same color to line the lashes on the upper lid only (C). Curl the lashes and finish with two coats of mascara on the upper lashes only, concentrating the mascara in the middle and outer corners of the eye using upward strokes. Use a flesh or white liner to line inside of lower lashes.

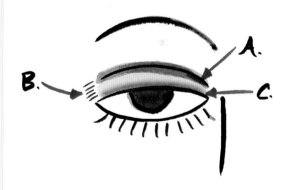

FOR CLOSE-SET EYES:

Like moving furniture around your house or apartment, the goal with close-set eyes is to give the illusion of more space (between the eyes). Use a lighter shade to the inner third of the lid from the lashes to the brow bone (A). Next, apply the dark shade to the outer two thirds of the eye from the lash line to the brow bone (B). Concentrate color on the far corners of your eyes, extending slightly past your natural line (C). Blend. Apply liner to only the outer third of the upper lash line (D). Apply mascara.

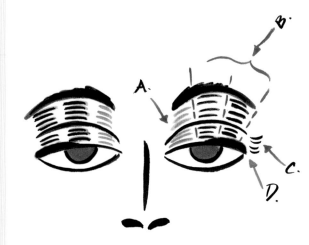

FOR WIDE-SET EYES:

The goal is to give the illusion of less space between the eyes. Just know that wide-set eyes are currently in vogue. Check out the current crop of models used by *Vogue* and other fashion magazines. But our goal is to make you look and feel great, so the hell with what they are dictating. This tutorial aims to make the space between them narrower. Begin by applying the lighter shade to the outer two thirds of the lid (A). Start at the lashes and blend upward, stopping at the brow bone. Next use the dark shade on the inside third of the eye, from the lash line to the brow bone and blend upward (B). Apply eyeliner from the inner to outer corner of the upper lid (C). Apply mascara.

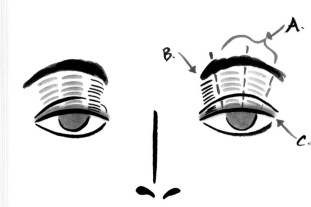

Now that we've had a few lessons in how to apply this trio of eye products, let's open our eyes to the simple truth about eye shadow, eyeliner, and mascara: Despite the ridiculous number of products and colors and blends out there vying for your attention and your wallet, if you keep it simple, you can't go wrong.

eye shadow

The truth is, all powders are pretty much equal. Powder products are tricky products to produce; it requires the right amount of milling and pressing to create a finely milled, soft, and blendable product. The equipment to do this is expensive, and there are key "outside" vendors that are able to do this with great expertise, thus, many of the big companies use these same few vendors to produce their shadows and then simply label it as their own. So it is hard to say one product is better than the other. Additionally, the same ingredients are generally used to create the base of the shadow, which generally contains talc, mica, ethylhexyl palmitate, zince stearate, methylparaben, propylparaben, and silica, plus added minerals and colorants to create the shade. One big difference, however, is that some of these powder eye shadows claim to

be made with minerals that are said to be less irritating and safer for the eye—but be forewarned, some people find these mineral products to be more irritating.

A word to the wise: Many "drugstore" brands use these same outside vendors for their eye shadow as higher-end brands, so see if they have your favorite shade in a finely milled and pressed powder before you drop a bundle for a shadow in places like Sephora, Nordstrom, or other higher-end retailers.

> A word to the wise: Many "drugstore" brands use these same outside vendors for their eye shadow as higher-end brands.

When it comes to color, what I've discovered since my eye-opening weekend with Mrs. X is that the best shadow duos are the beige to brown for dark eyes, or the gray to black family for light eyes. One or both of these shadow families will look good and appropriate on everyone. Unless you want to look like a peacock, forget the plums and pinks, greens and blues. Neutral tones are more natural, letting your eyes do the magic. Leave the garish look for Halloween. And much like my rule for lipstick colors, your eye shadow should not contain high levels of metallics, shimmer, and glitter. Dark shades combined with lighter neutrals are the most forgiving and youthful choices for the lids.

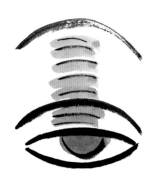

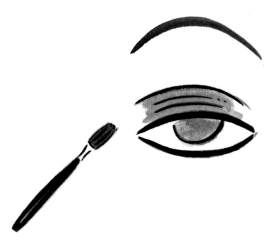

HERE ARE A FEW BEST BETS:

Singles:

- CoverGirl Eye Enhancers 1 Kit Shadow: Brown Smolder and Swiss Chocolate
- L'Oreal Paris Studio Secrets Professional Eye Shadow Singles in Lush Raven
- Lancôme Color Design Singles: Mochaccino and Colour du Jour
- Nars Single Eye Shadow: Fez and Coconut Grove
- Trish McEvoy Eye Shadow: Soft Grey and Glamorous
- Giorgio Armani Eyes to Kill Eyeshadow: #1 and #6

Duos:

- Clinique All About Shadow Duo in Like Mink
- Maybelline Expert Wear Duo Eye Shadow in Browntones
- Kevyn Aucoin Eyeshadow Duo in #207 Soft Gold Lame/Smokey Brown

eyeliner

Eyeliner does for the eyes what a good accessory does for clothes: It enhances and completes the look. What would Chanel suits be without gold chains and pearls? Good, but much more FABULOUS with them. Some women depend on eyeliner to change the shape of their eyes, while others value the way it seems to open the eyes and draw attention to make them appear bigger. In either case, used properly, eyeliner is a great asset.

That said, there are only a few occasions when I will say NEVER in this book, and this is one: Never ever use a liquid liner—it looks hard and emphasizes the delicate (often crêpe-y) and fine skin surrounding your eyes. Soft pencil liners (that can be smudged) are my preferred form because of their manageability. Powder liner will work as well, but they tend to flake and leave a mess under the eyes, requiring additional cleanup. Here, too, neutrals work best. The bright blues, purples, and greens are best to put on hold . . . forever.

MY PICK OF BEST BETS:

- CoverGirl Perfect Blend Eyeliner
- Elizabeth Arden Beautiful Color Smoky Eyes
- MAC Eye Kohl

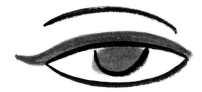

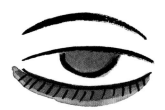

mascara

When it comes to makeup, mascara is always a subject of great interest to women: Who among us wouldn't love to have long, thick, voluminous, beautiful lashes? As we get older, however, our lashes become sparse, making it more difficult to create the look that we once had. But don't get caught up in the mascara hype. Claims like "400 percent more volumized," or "100 times thicker," or "extreme-length" have to be taken with a grain of salt. Instead, experiment with a formula and brush that covers the "grays" and combs through *your* lashes, making them look the most natural, well-defined, and clumpless. Trying to create more lashes with unreasonable expectations from your mascara will most likely create more of a problem than a solution. There are a few go-to mascaras that work extremely well for the average set of lashes, so it might be helpful to start with the following **Best Bets**:

- CoverGirl LashBlast Volume Mascara

- CoverGirl LashBlast Clump Crusher

- L'Oreal Paris Voluminous Original Mascara

- Lancôme Définicils

Most everyday formulas wear well throughout the day without smudging and are easily removable with soap and water or simple eye makeup remover. These are your best bets. Avoid regular use of waterproof formulas. Save those for special occasions, like tears at your daughter's wedding. They are too tough to remove for everyday use—you'll have to rub hard to loosen the color, and in doing so you risk breaking your fragile lashes.

makeup tools

Never underestimate the power of a good tool to get the job done. Thankfully, we don't need anything complicated or hard to operate—just a few brushes and other simple applicators. While some products, like eye shadows and powder liners, often come with their own application brush, they're generally poorly made, not the right size, and difficult to hold. It's worth investing a few dollars in high-quality makeup tools to, yes, get the job done—and well.

PRIMER SPONGE

In lieu of your finger, a well-shaped sponge works wonders at reaching the tight spots around the eyes and nose.

A few **Best Bets:**
- Beauty Blender (these are allergen and latex-free, with no harsh chemicals)
- Sephora Collection The Perfectionist Makeup Sponge

BRUSHES

You might be surprised to know that the material of your brush plays a role in the quality of your makeup application. The makeup formulas you use will help you determine whether to choose natural (real) or synthetic (fake) hair. Natural brushes are better for dry products like blush and eye shadow, and synthetic brushes are best suited for cream or liquid because they soak up less formula than natural hair.

To keep them clean and to avoid bacteria build-up, wash with soap and water (or baby shampoo) one or more times a week and air dry on a clean towel. Since buying a good set of brushes will set you back a hefty sum, be careful not to let water touch the shank of the brush where the hairs are held together, otherwise the metal will rust and the brush will start to disintegrate.

Shadow Brush

Use a flat, round-tip, natural-hair brush that is firm enough to pick up the shadow yet soft enough to spread it gently without being harsh to our delicate lids. Pony and goat hair brushes don't shed and give a precise application.

Best Bets:
- Sephora Pro Shadow Brush #14
- Trish McEvoy Brush 45

Angled Eyeliner Brush

Use a slim, tapered, synthetic, firm-bristled brush. The hairs should be tightly packed and have a sharp-angled straight edge so they can, with some precision, distribute the dark color along the lash line, and into an up-and-out direction.

Best Bets:
- Benefit Hard Angled Definer Brush
- Trish McEvoy Brush 50
- e.l.f. Studio Angled Eyeliner Brush

Thin Eyeliner Smudge Brush

Use a flat, short-haired brush with a rounded tip that is dense and tightly enough packed to pick up the shadow color and distribute it along the lash line with soft, smooth strokes. These brushes do a great job in softening the look of eyeliner.

Best Bets:

- Jane Iredale Smudge Brush
- NARS Smudging Brush
- Trish McEvoy Va Va Voom Smudge Brush 54

DUAL ENDED Q-TIPS

These old-school bathroom staples do an exceptional job at doing double-duty as makeup applicators. Use the pointed end to pick up highlighter or concealer to place under the outer edge of the shadow and on the inside corner of the eye. Only a dot is needed. Blend with the rounded corner of the Q-tip.

EYELASH CURLER

Last but not least, I want to mention the value of a good eyelash curler. It opens up the eyes, making them look bigger, wider, and brighter, and these are extremely valuable qualities as we cut back on the heavier eye makeup we most likely used in the past. To avoid eyelash breakage, curl the lashes *first*, gently and close to the root, and then apply mascara. Be sure you use a good curler with a comfortable grip and a high-quality rubber piece.

Best Bets:

- Kevyn Aucoin The Eyelash Curler
- Maybelline Expert Tools Eyelash Curler
- Sally Hansen Flirty Eyes Classic Eyelash Curler
- Shu Uemura Eyelash Curler

only a dot is needed . . .

bad hair days

During and after menopause, thinning hair often becomes a concern. Turns out, our declining estrogen levels don't just affect the hair on our heads; our lashes and brows also tend to thin and gray as we age. While all mascaras will cover gray and help mask thinning lashes, there may come a time when mascara alone won't suffice in making so-so lashes look super. The good news is that when lashes thin out or break, or there's simply not enough hair to coat evenly with mascara, there are many weapons you can do battle with, relative to your cosmetic regimen.

FALSE EYELASHES

Having supervised so many editorial and ad campaigns throughout my career, I always appreciated what false eyelashes did to a model or celebrity for the camera, but I never put much stock in wearing them for real life, despite the influence of Liza and Twiggy. Tammy Faye kind of put the kibosh on that one—that is, until my friend Gloria showed me her eyelash technique, which came in handy when she had chemo and lost all her hair! So here are Gloria's foolproof steps for buying and wearing false lashes that look undetectably natural, with or without your own lash hair:

1 Shop at the drugstore and pay no more than $2.99 a pair for real hair lashes. Gloria's favorite brand for the most natural-looking lashes is Andrea #53, and for a little more fullness, Elite #18. Buy a few at a time because stock runs out on these two favorites.

2 Unless you wear brown mascara, look for black lashes.

3 Buy a tube of dark Duo Adhesive and a box of toothpicks.

4 When you get home, take them out of the box gently and lay them along your lash line (this step is essential whether you have lashes or not).

5 Invariably, they will be too wide for your eyelid, and you will have to cut them from the longer lash side to fit your lid.

6 Save the lashes you've trimmed. You'll need them later.

7 Before proceeding, put your eye makeup on. If you have lashes, apply one thin coat of mascara (before using the false lashes) to establish a good base.

8 Squeeze a miniscule dot of Duo adhesive on the top of your hand. Dab the tip of a toothpick into the Duo and apply a very thin layer along the base of the false lash strip. Wait about 30 seconds, then apply to your own lash line. Work from the outer corner in. Gently press with ring finer to set the lashes in place.

9 For fuller day lashes or for evening wear, take the lashes you've just trimmed off and apply them to the outer corner of the eye on top of the already applied lashes, using the same glue technique. If you are lucky enough to have fairly full lashes, use these trimmed pieces for daily use on the outer edges of the eye and use the full strip for evening.

10 Keep the tube of Duo and a toothpick in your cosmetic pouch for a quick touchup, should one of your lashes detach.

Like your first week of yoga classes, the first few times you try to apply false eyelashes can prove daunting, but, with a little practice, you'll become a pro. And don't worry, you will never look like Tammy Faye or Ru Paul with this routine. This is one of those moments when less (your lashes) is really more (with false lashes), in terms of its benefits. A pair of lashes should last at least a week if you remove them gently each night, take off the adhesive with your fingertips, and place them back on the form they came with.

EYELASH EXTENSIONS

A lot of women use eyelash extensions, but be aware that, while they are attractive, the procedure is time-consuming and costly (between $50–$100 for the initial application) and maintenance is required every three weeks. Like hair extensions, there are risks to using them, and, when not applied properly, it puts one's natural lash in danger of falling out or breaking off—even permanent loss of hair. And like hair extensions, the long thick lashes can be addictive. When Gloria's eyelashes were growing back after chemo, she was advised by the extension technician to continue using false eyelashes, since her own lashes were too weak for extensions at that stage of growth. Now, even though she's a candidate for extensions, she's happy to stick with her false eyelashes. She's perfected the method, taking only a minute per eye to apply them, avoiding the expense and time involved in getting extensions.

Having said all of this, here are a few vital pieces of information to know if you decide to pursue extensions:

- Do your research. Go to a reputable salon (preferably one recommended and tried by friends). Consider having a free consultation first, and, while there, check to be certain the lash artist is a licensed aesthetician or cosmetologist.

- Be sure the technician is not applying "cluster lash" extensions. It should be one single lash applied to each one of your own lashes.

- Avoid getting the extensions wet for 24 to 48 hours after application. The adhesive will reactivate and may cause the lashes to stick together and look like caked-on mascara.

- Don't touch! No pulling, tugging, or twisting. You can damage your lashes or even your lids. Don't try to remove them yourself; always have them professionally removed.

- Stay away from oil-based and moisture-rich hair products and face creams—they will loosen the bond. When washing hair, tilt head back.

EYELASH TINTING

This procedure, which is more affordable than extensions (from $15–$50 dollars), works best if you have lots of lashes, very light lashes (blond, red, or gray), and/or light tips on your natural lashes. You can achieve spectacular eye definition with lash tinting, allowing you to skip wearing mascara all together, but don't expect longer or thicker lashes—only darker and more defined lashes. To maintain your tint, you should have your lashes retouched every four to six weeks, but it only takes thirty minutes in a salon. I am a convert and regular user for many years, and here's what I've learned:

- Never use DIY, at-home products; you risk eye infections and irritation. It's always great to save money, but your eyes are important and delicate—treat them as a precious investment.

- Before tinting, research the salon's reputation, and the skill and experience of the aesthetician.

- Be sure to do an allergy and sensitivity patch test *before* making a commitment.

- Have some saline or lubricating solution to apply after the treatment (my aesthetician supplies a generous dose of this at the end of the treatment).

- Black is by far the most effective tint color, as it really makes lashes stand out.

ALERT: Eyelash tinting may be illegal in your state because there is a history of irritation caused by the misuse of coal-tar dyes on the lashes. Never allow your eyelashes to be tinted with anything other than vegetable-based dyes.

EYELASH GROWTH TREATMENTS

If you have thinning or short lashes, and you want longer, fuller lashes that don't require upkeep, you should know about Latisse, which is an FDA-approved, prescription-only drug (originally used for treatment of glaucoma and ocular pressure). It is by no means a perfect solution because, while it effectively enhances lash thickness and length of lashes, Latisse does have proven downsides: In some patients, the drug company reported a permanent brown pigmentation of the iris and eyelid skin darkening, as well as redness, itchiness, and dry eye. So be forewarned, and take my advice: consider safer, over-the-counter products that condition the lashes and provide moisture and shine.

Best Bets:
- RapidLash Eyelash & Eyebrow Enhancing Serum
- Prevage Clinical Lash and Brow Enhancing Serum

eyebrows

Have you ever noticed how downturned eyes are often accompanied by downturned brows? This "pairing" can often age a face, but a well-groomed brow can be a subtle and effective way to enhance the eyes and give your face a more youthful expression. Like a picture frame enhances a painting, the brow draws attention to your eyes. Fuller, more natural, brows give a youthful look, and well-shaped brows open up your face, bringing out bone structure and giving eyes the illusion of being bigger than they actually are. Groomed brows add definition to eyes, and it should be considered a key step in your makeup regimen.

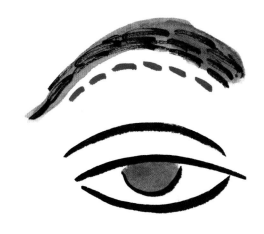

EYEBROW SHAPING

While many of us are adept at plucking our own brows, I highly recommend leaving this important grooming technique to a professional. Even if you ultimately want to be in control of your own brows, it is helpful to get started with a good professional. Once the shape is determined and set, you can easily maintain them, leaving less of a margin for haphazard plucking errors.

Droopy eyes can be changed by slightly arching the brows and extending them outward toward the temples (rather than having the tail curve down around the eye). The arch is an important part of the brow and should be a gradual and very gentle lift in line with the outer third of the eye.

The three standard techniques for shaping are tweezing, waxing, or threading (a salon method of hair removal with a thread). I say choose the method that hurts you the least! I prefer the speedy, at-home maintenance of tweezing, but the key takeaway here is that groomed, well-shaped brows are as crucial as eye makeup for a youthful appearance. Yes, taking care of your brows is that important.

BROW COLOR

Brows should never be lighter than your hair color. This dulls the face and gives a pale pallor to your complexion. The brows can be up to two shades darker than your hair, but, if you are using a pencil to fill in some missing brow hair, choose a shade lighter than your eyebrow hair color, otherwise it will look fake. Use short light strokes to fill in the gaps, and extend the outer ends just beyond the eyes. For a natural look, try dual-ended pencils that give you the choice of blending two colors together.

If you have patchy spots, another option is to use a brow powder. Just make sure the outer edges of the brows don't disappear. The tail of the brow is important, as it creates the youthful outward direction for the brow and gives some emphasis to the arch, but it should never be a hard, dark line. What about gray brows? Never ever pluck. Not even one stray. Hide gray strays either by dyeing at your local hair colorist, spa, or brow bar, or by using a brow marker. The felt-tip point lets you paint hairs precisely. You can also use a mascara-type "brow tint" to help camouflage all the grays (see below).

Best Bets:
- Benefit Brow Zing (eyebrow powder)
- Lancôme's Le Crayon Poudre Powder Pencil
- Milani Brow Tint Pen
- Paula Dorf Brow Tint
- TouchBack Brow Marker

the tail of the brow is important . . .

WHILE I MAY never reveal the identity of the fabulous Mrs. X, I am thrilled to spill the details of her eye makeup regimen. Learning it was a game changer for me, and not just because she taught me a quick and foolproof cosmetic routine for my eyes. More important, she taught me the power of the eyes, not only to seduce and flirt, but also to see and to learn, to embrace and to enhance, what we've been given. She was undaunted by crow's feet, unalarmed by wrinkles, undiscouraged by dark circles, and unflinching when it came to taking hold of her talents—in this case her eyes—and using them to the max. And now that you know her secret, why shouldn't you take advantage of it, too?

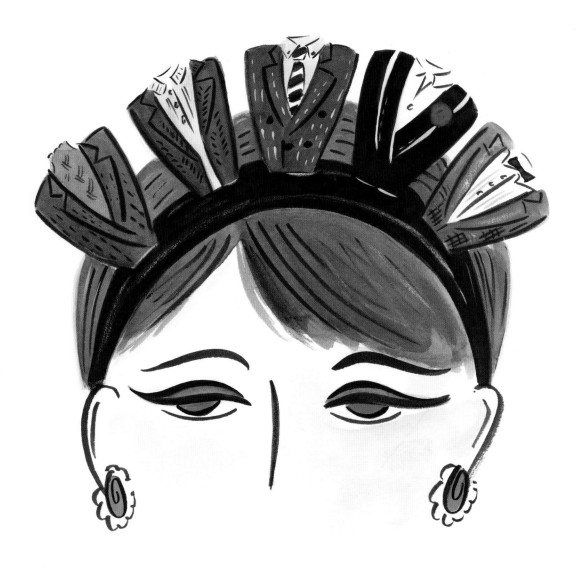

In a hurry but don't want naked lids? Skip the eye shadow routine and just use a natural shade primer on your lids, followed by a soft line of dark shadow along the upper and lower lashes. Or use a soft eye pencil in a dark shade, smudging it along the lash line in the same upward and outward direction.

If you are in a *real* hurry, mix primer and concealer to diffuse lines and wrinkles on your eyelids, then finish with mascara.

If you're like me and have very heavy brows with rogue hairs, here's a great trick to keeping them looking neat and groomed, which I learned from Kevyn Aucoin. Brush all your brow hairs up using a spoolie brush, then use brow scissors to cut the tips of the hairs that extend above the top of the brow. Tweezerman Brow Shaping Scissors are one of the best tools to use for this purpose. Their slanted, stainless-steel tip firmly grips hair at the base so that you can ease them out without pinching. They are light and easy to handle and come in bright colors, making them easy to find in your makeup bag. Another added bonus: Your Tweezerman comes with a lifetime guarantee and free sharpening.

MASCARA WARS

A little inside "dirt" is always fun to know. L'Oreal Paris and CoverGirl are long-time rivals in many cosmetics areas, but none so competitively as mascara. L'Oreal has been the all-time leader in the category for well over twenty years, and here is how they did it. They had a particular gentleman in their product development department who invented all their mascara brushes and developed winner after winner that was immediately patented so that competitors could not copy or imitate these designs (or "masterpieces," in the world of cosmetics). This mascara master would come to meetings that I attended with a briefcase full of his latest designs and pull out a mirror and demonstrate on his *own* lashes the benefit of each new brush he had invented. Many cosmetics companies tried to invent competitive products, but L'Oreal held the leading edge—and the patents—on the designs, thereby blocking the competition. That is, until CoverGirl invented the big, orange, molded plastic brush which became an overnight winner with CoverGirl LashBlast, breaking the L'Oreal winning streak and starting the legendary "Mascara Wars." And they are still duking it out today, with every new mascara launch.

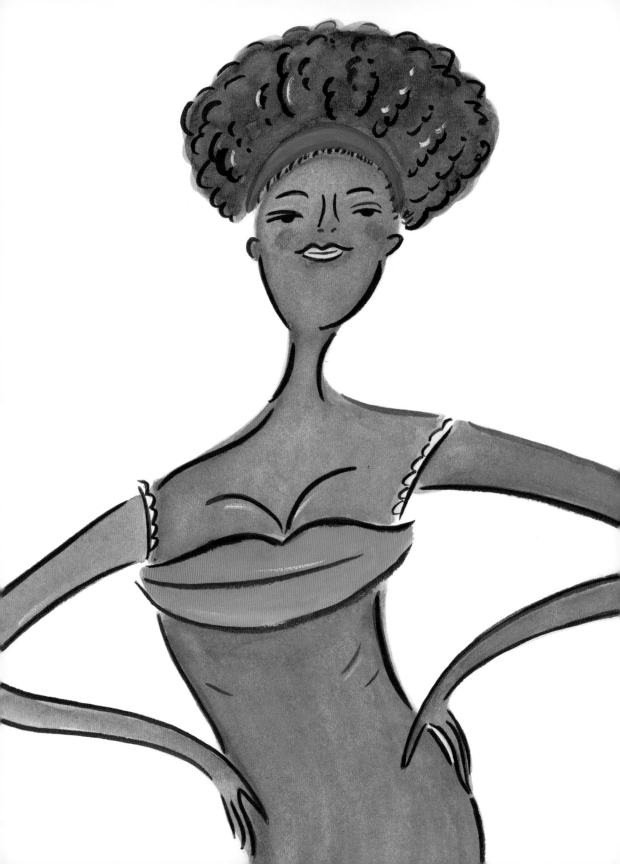

CHAPTER NINE

Lipstick

the magic bullet

IT'S TIME TO GET RID OF THOSE STICKY, TACKY, HIGH-SHINE, LACQUERED TUBES. SIMPLY PUT: TOSS THE GLOSS.

If foundation is the perfect white T-shirt of your cosmetic bag, then lipstick is the push-up bra, giving you added sex appeal, and radiating sophistication and confidence. But let me be clear: I'm talking lipstick, not lip gloss.

If you're one of the millions of women who've hit fifty and think gloss is the answer to fabulous lips, boy am I glad that we've found each other. If you have those nasty little vertical demon lines above your upper lip, you can't use it anymore. Sorry. The same thing goes for all dark lipsticks. See also: red lipstick. Unless you have rich dark skin or plump lineless lips, toss those deep shades. They may seem sexy and sophisticated in the tube, but dark shades creep into those lines around your mouth and nothing ages you more than "bleeding" lipstick. I know this seems counterintuitive. You're embracing your sexuality, your confidence, and your inner goddess, and you have to renounce

It's time to take those sticky, tacky, lacquered tubes of high gloss and shine and toss them out!

the very makeup item that symbolizes all of that. I feel your pain. I remember how great that little black dress looked on my thirtieth birthday, wearing nothing else but my red lips. I remember "Cherries in the Snow" and "Fire and Ice" and that rush of sexual confidence that came from swiping a bit of red on my lips before a date with Mr. Guess Who.

But if you want to look good now, wearing red lipstick will kill your game. It looks like you're trying too hard—there are other ways to exude sex appeal. BUT—that doesn't mean we have to forget about our mouths and call it a day. Au contraire . . .

Neutral is the new name of the game. The right shade of neutral can compensate and draw attention away from our less-attractive features, while red lipstick or very dark shades can emphasize dark circles under the eyes and make your lips look thin. Whether it's a silky taupe, creamy caramel, nude pink, dusty fawn, or light chocolate, it's time to embrace neutral lipstick and learn how to work our most feminine feature in a different way.

It all goes back to my twelve-year-old memory of Tangee. Remember that lipstick? It was orange in the stick, but, as you put it on, your mouth was magically transformed into the most perfect shade of "lip"—not orange at all, but a rosy, natural shade that somehow gave my adolescent lips a luscious, smooth, naturally-tinted fullness that transported me into the world of

i was hooked . . .

sophisticated women. I was hooked, and so was every boy on my street—I kissed them all that summer. This was the beginning of my love affair with subtle naked lip shades.

Many of us will remember when it was nearly impossible to find a good neutral shade. That's why, as I mentioned in the opening of the book, I created The Nakeds and The Naughty Nakeds when I was president of Ultima II. Since I am the quintessential au naturel "babe" at heart, I wanted to create a group of neutral lip colors that were good for women of all ethnicities, a group of colors that spoke up for our deepest beauty instincts, a group of colors that shouted, "This is who we are!" Now more than ever, with the confidence and wisdom of experience and the arsenal of beauty info I'll supply, we are going to enjoy looking like ourselves, only better. To loosely paraphrase Gloria Steinem, "This is what 50, 60, 70, 80, 90 looks like, and it's pretty damn good."

This chapter is about the seduction of that magic shade range, and how your lips can be just as powerful, compelling, and sexy with neutrals as they were with bright reds and pinks. Getting the lips right can give the entire face a more youthful appearance. After all, at a time of life when you have a lot to say, why not call some extra attention to your mouth.

drawing the line with lip shaping

Let's start with an indispensible tool—lip liner—and learn how to build a fabulous mouth. Personally, I am an ardent and faithful devotee of lip pencils. I would even choose one over straight-up lipstick, because with a good lip pencil I can create (draw) the mouth I want, and then add lip balm to make them look moist and plump. Be sure to select a neutral matte pencil (wood-clenched is best, where the color is imbedded in the wood, just like in a lead pencil), and choose a shade that's close to your natural lip color.

Sharpen the pencil (the line must be very thin and fine). Use the pencil to draw a line just above the outside edge of your natural lip line. If you can't see your lip line any more (as we age, many of us lose our lips or our lips become very thin), get out some old pictures of yourself that you like, and, with the help of a magnifying mirror, try to imitate the natural line of the mouth you once had. This requires practice, so don't get frustrated if your lips aren't perfect right away.

If your lip line has faded, follow this simple ten-step process to redefine your lips. Practice makes perfect!

1 Place your index finger vertically under one of your nostrils (right nostril with right hand, left with left hand), with your fingertip resting just beneath the nostril opening.

2 With the lip liner pencil, place one dot on the upper lip area aligning the dot on the inside edge of your finger next to the first joint of your finger.

3 Repeat with the other hand and nostril. Draw a short vertical line in the middle of the two dots on the upper lip (it should be a bit shorter than the height of the two dots).

4 Next, starting on one side of your mouth, draw a line from the outside corner of your mouth, up to the dot on your upper lip area.

5 Repeat on the other side.

6 Draw a diagonal line down from each dot to the top of a short vertical line in the middle of the dots. This forms the peaks of the upper lip.

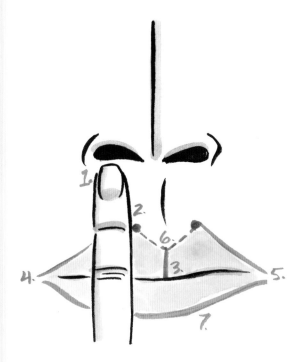

7 Line the outside of the lower lips, since it is most often the upper lip that disappears.

8 Once you like what you see, fill in the lips with the lip liner and take a picture with your phone. (When I am unsure about a piece of makeup I've used—or even a new hairstyle—I always take a picture. It's better than looking in the mirror where one can lose perspective.)

9 Last, apply your lipstick. Start in the middle of your lips to avoid color clumping at the corners of the mouth. I usually just swipe it on hurriedly from the tube, but, when I really want to look good, I go the extra distance and use a lip brush. (See sidebar for information on lip brushes.)

And that's it! Just make sure that the lip line you created is lightly covered with lip color, as is the rest of your mouth. You want to avoid the look of a heavy lip liner at all costs.

HERE ARE A FEW OF MY FAVORITE LINERS:

- Chanel Precision Lip Definer in Mordore-Nude (a creamy, midtone brown liner that comes with its own sharpener)
- L'Oreal Colour Riche Lip Liner in Au Naturale and Forever Rose (neutral enough to work with many shades in the neutral palette)
- MAC Cosmetics Lip Pencil in Spice or Stripdown (looks great on everybody and blends well with virtually any shade of neutral)

inside the lines

Now that you've mastered the art of lining your lips, it's time to focus on the finishing touch: lipstick. Depending on your lip shape and condition, sometimes lipstick is all you need. But now that traditional darks most likely no longer do it, how do we determine the best color for our skin tone and coloring? And what about texture and wear? Like most cosmetics, the "choice effect" with lipsticks can leave us paralyzed when it comes to choosing the appropriate products. There are just too many to select from. Often, we default to our tried-and-true colors and brands, but, as our skin color changes through the years, these colors and styles may no longer suit our needs. Additionally, it's important to know the inside scoop on the labels and formulas before investing in lip products. Remember how I mentioned before that makeup and skincare formulas for the large cosmetic corporations are most often developed in a central research and development laboratory that services all divisions or brands in the corporation? The same applies here. So be aware of the following: A few years ago, a lipstick breakthrough formula would have first been applied to the most upscale brand of all the divisions. The theory behind this was that a brand like Lancôme (sold at department stores) was the most prestigious and fashion-forward brand, so Lancôme might get the technology first, and then, for example, L'Oreal Paris (sold in drugstores) might utilize the same technology some period of time after that. The cosmetic industry called this the "trickle down" effect. In other words, the customers who shopped for high-end brands were thought to be the most fashion-forward, and they bought their products in department stores. By selling these "high-end" brands at department stores, companies ensured their prestige status. Later in the shopping cycle, the wisdom went, that style preference would "trickle down" to the less fashionable drugstore shoppers. But consumer behaviors changed, as did the market, and cosmetics corporations soon discovered that time-starved women (often raising a family and holding down a job at the same time) began cross-shopping in drugstores and anywhere else she could meet her beauty and shopping needs, thereby diluting the high-end market. Today, corporations are more likely to give new lipstick formulas to their lower-end brands first! And by the way, the lower-end brands have stepped up their fashion quotient dramatically over the last decade. The lesson: Don't be fooled by fancy packaging and shade names—you may very well find the same formula in less expensive brands. So check at CVS first!

LIPSTICK SHADE

Finding the right lip color can be tricky, so use the following guide to help you select the neutral color family that will look most flattering:

Fair or Pale Skin Tones

Look for neutrals with soft pinks, pale peaches, and apricot undertones and avoid beige lipstick that can wash you out.

Here are your **Best Bets:**
- NARS Dolce Vita, Barbarella
- Revlon Super Lustrous Lipstick in Demure
- Rimmel London Moisture Renew Lip Colour in To Nude or Not to Nude

Golden Skin Tones

Go for creamy, caramel, and clay-toned nudes and warm beiges. If your skin is deeper, look for midtone beige, like mocha and rich latte. Avoid anything cool in undertone, like mauve.

Consider these **Best Bets:**
- Chanel Rouge Coco Shine in Boy
- Dior Rouge Dior Lip Color in Trompe L'Oeil
- L'Oreal Paris Colour Riche Lip Color in Gilded Pink

- Maybelline Color Sensational Lip Color in Warm Me Up

Olive Skin Tones

If your skin is deeper than golden, but not dark, look for midtone beiges like mocha and rich latte. Avoid anything cool in undertone, like mauve. The Tom Ford recommendation below hits the right amount of beige without going too dark.

Best Bets:
- Maybelline's Color Sensational Lipcolor in Totally Toffee
- Nuance Salma Hayek Color Vibrance Lipstick in Nude
- Sonia Kashuk Satin Luxe Lipcolor with SPF 16 in Barely Nude
- Tom Ford Lip Color in Sable Smoke

Dark Skin Tones

Opt for chocolate tones, such as rich golden-browns like coffee, and avoid anything remotely orange as it makes skin look drab.

Best Bets:

- CoverGirl Coloricious Lipstick in Tempting Toffee 255
- CoverGirl Queen Collection Lipcolor in Coffee Break
- Laura Mercier Crème Smooth Lip Colour in Cocoa and Dulce de Leche
- Wet 'N Wild Mega Shield Lip Color SPF 15 in Bare-ly Legal

LIPSTICK TEXTURE

Now let's discuss texture, since the right texture choice is the make-or-break factor on your mouth. The three most common choices are matte, frost or shimmers, and creamy/shine. Here's the low-down on the pros and cons of each:

Matte

Want to look really old? No? Then run away from this pasty, drying look as fast as you can.

Frost

Want to look really cheap? No? Then if you move to shimmer, make it very subtle, or prepare to resemble Blanche from *The Golden Girls*.

Creamy/Shine

Ding, ding, ding! You've found the winner! Rich, moist-looking lips that make your mouth look full and soft, satiny and youthful. Forget about high gloss, metallics, and glitter—save those for costume parties only.

Best Bets worth considering:

- CoverGirl Coloricious Lipstick in Dulce de Léche 225, Caramel Kiss 240 and Tempting Toffee 255
- Dolce and Gabbana Classic Cream Lipstick in Petal, Mandorla, and Cashmere
- Maybelline New York Color Sensational Lip Color in Born With It, Nearly There, and Totally Toffee
- N.Y.C. Ultra Moist Lipwear in Petal, Chiffon, and Mocha

Now that you've narrowed your choices down to shade and texture, here are a few insider tips to help your lip color look even better:

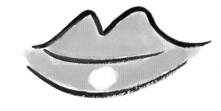

- For a fuller mouth, dab the slightest bit of Vaseline or shiny moisturizing lip balm (don't buy lip gloss) on the middle of the lower lip.

- For a fuller upper-lip look, dot highlighter between the peaks of the lips (the Cupid's bow).

- When choosing between two colors, opt for the lighter one. Pale colors make lips look fuller.

- For a longer-lasting color, avoid using matte lipsticks and use instead a lip stain before applying lipstick.

- For a longer-lasting color, apply lipstick straight from the tube, blot with a tissue and apply the lipstick again. The second swipe will also add shine and coverage

- Before using your lip liner, cover your lips with foundation, concealer, or primer—this will also help the color last.

- To avoid hard edges, roll the tip of your lip liner around on the palm of your hand before using.

- If you've made a mistake and your lips are too dark, gently blend in some foundation or concealer to lighten them.

- Test lip color in the store on your fingertip— not the side of your hand!—as that is closest to your natural lip shade.

ALL DAY LIPSTICKS

No one knows more about the birth of this category than I do since it was invented by my team at Revlon's Ultima II when I was president. The first product entry in the market was called LipSexxxy. This category caused a minor sensation in the marketplace, especially with working women, who wanted to have lipstick that they didn't have to apply during the day, that didn't come off on drinking glasses, and that didn't come off on fabric. The lipsticks flew off the store shelves and our competitors rushed to copy us. The tradeoff compared to regular lipsticks on the market was that they were rather dry on the lips. Since then, several companies, including Revlon, have come up with liquid lipsticks that are available in intense pigments with long-lasting polymers and moisturizing ingredients like vitamin E and argan oil to keep lips hydrated.

Consider these **Best Bets:**
- e.l.f. Essential Luscious Liquid Lipstick in Maple Sugar
- Hourglass Opaque Rouge Liquid Lipstick in Canvas
- Revlon ColorStay Ultimate Liquid Lipstick in Nude
- Yves Saint Laurent Rouge Pur Couture Vernis à Lèvres Glossy Stain in Beige Aquarelle

And while we're on the subject of hydration, one of the best sources for great-looking, super-hydrated lips without having to resort to lip gloss is tinted lip balm. Not only do they come in lip-enhancing natural shades that soothe and condition, but some also come with a sun protection factor.

Try these **Best Bets:**
- Burt's Bees Tinted Lip Balm in Caramel
- Clinique Chubby Sticks Moisturizing Lip Colour Balm in Curvy Candy
- Maybelline New York Baby Lips Moisturizing Lip Balm in Peach Kiss

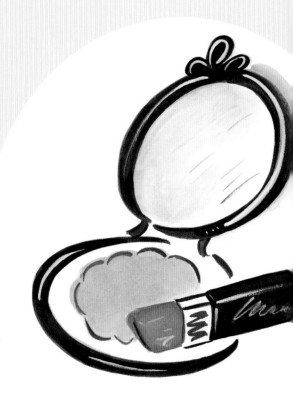

lip rehab

Our lips aren't always fit for color. In fact, sometimes they need serious intervention before color even comes in to the picture. Weather, neglect, age, even illness can wreak havoc on our soft-skinned kissers.

If your lips look anything like mine have looked on occasion—cracked, wrinkled, chapped—they need a good stint of therapy. Sometimes, they require a little help to spring back to the sexy little place they once held on your face. Here's what to do:

EXFOLIATE

Yes, you can—and should—exfoliate your lips. They, too, get dead-skin buildup. Getting rid of all the dead cells will make your lips look smoother and plumper and help foster new cell turnover. If they're chapped, a quick, soothing, and effective at-home remedy for ridding your lips of the flaky bits of skin you're so tempted to chew off is to hold a warm, wet washcloth (with texture) against them for a couple of minutes, then rub the washcloth (or a soft toothbrush) in a circular motion to gently slough off the moistened dead skin. Follow up by coating them with a good lip balm with SPF. I suggest avoiding commercial lip plumpers, as they irritate the skin for none to minimal results. Instead, just keep lips hydrated. And NEVER lick your lips to moisten them, especially in windy conditions! Though it may alleviate dryness in the moment, it's like drinking saltwater when you're thirsty: It

just dries them out further. There are a number of good lip balms and exfoliants on the market. Some **Best Bets:**

- Aquaphor Lip Repair and Protect SPF 30
- Bliss Fabulips Sugar Lip Scrub
- Fresh Sugar Lip Polish

It's also worth noting that good old-fashioned Carmex does the trick, as does Vaseline—both excellent agents for dry lips. We often get so used to using a lip balm when our lips are chapped that when we stop using it we have the sensation that our lips have dried out. After several days of using lip balm, it's better to ease off and get back to our regular moisturizing lipstick.

Now, let's "chew the fat" about more permanent solutions for problems like disappearing lips and those nasty vertical lines that plague our upper lips.

LIP INJECTIONS

Lips gone entirely? In this case, if your budget can afford it, I would opt for help from a good dermatologist. The operative words here are "good" (someone with proven skills on this part of the face) and "budget" (it's expensive). You certainly don't want to end up with "trout pouts" like Lisa Rinna (she just had hers corrected, at great expense) or Goldie Hawn in *The First Wives Club*. You need a reputable expert who will build up your mouth gradually, using Restylane or Juvaderm (both hyluronic acids). This is a very precarious undertaking, one that can easily go awry in the hands of a doctor who lacks experience or a good eye. You can end up with much-too-much (the Angelina Jolie look on steroids) or not enough (a big waste of your money). Dr. Gervaise Gerstner, a well-known board-certified New York dermatologist and expert in the world of fillers, has saved many faces by injecting lips that have all but disappeared.

When is it worth considering this procedure? When the upper lip has rolled inward and is disproportionate to the lower lip. Dr. Gerstner's guideline for the "ideal size ratio of lips should be ⅓ top lip versus ⅔ bottom lip." She adds that patients should know that "lip filler doesn't last as long as filler lasts in other areas of the face,

as we use the lips so much." What does she use to battle the tiny little lines above the lip that cosmetics have a difficult time camouflaging? She favors a filler called Belotero.

Warning: Lip injections in the wrong hands are very obvious. An over-inflated mouth, and the little curl or roll back on the edge of the lips, is the dead giveaway. It has ruined the face of many a starlet, celebrity, and average Joe, so buyer beware. If your lips are merely thin, I would simply employ the less-permanent cosmetic remedies outlined above. As with any cosmetic surgery, there are downsides to lip injections:

- It hurts (while it's being injected)

- It's temporary (lasts three to six months)

- It will cost $500–$975 (the latter when two tubes of filler are used)

- You could end up with bruises that take days to go away

WRINKLE REMOVERS

Lip wrinkles are real demons. Once you notice these little vertical lines begin to appear along your upper lip line, they seem to turn into grooves and craters overnight! That said, I truly believe that they come from a life well-lived—a lot of smiling, talking with emotion, eating good food, drinking good wine, and generally lots of fun. But we are not going to let them have their way with us, are we? Here's what can be done.

Start by using moisturizers around the lips. Extra moisture can temporarily plump the skin and make the lines much less noticeable. Retin A and Renova work quite effectively in areas prone to wrinkles, like the eye and mouth area, but they are prescription-only and take several weeks to months to notice a softening of the lines.

Deeper lines can best be addressed by fractional lasers, dermabrasion, chemical peels, and fillers (Restylane and Juvaderm), Botox (the latter should be used with great care as there are many downsides, including drooping mouth and impaired speech), and Dr. Gerstner's favorite for this part of the face, too—Belotero. My advice? Avoid Botox on this area of the face, and go with one of the other technological advances I've mentioned instead—but bring your wallet. Like fillers for the lips, it is an expensive proposition ($500–$800). I have a friend who ended up in the hands of the wrong dermatologist when she was searching for a solution to her deepening lines above her mouth. She looked like she had an enlarged monkey mouth by the time he got through with her. He injected too much filler, and it took her six months to start looking halfway "normal" again. Lasers and microdermabrasion (for less severe lines) can be very effective, but be prepared for downtime and discomfort. I have another friend who opted for a very strong laser solution, and she was out of commission for over two weeks—a severe burn, painkillers, face bandages, peeling skin, and a Michael Jackson–type mask covering nose to chin. But the outcome, in her words, was "spectacular," and she would do it again if necessary. The result was that good. But it, too, is costly ($2,500).

Ultimately, your doctor will determine which laser procedure, chemical solution, or filler is appropriate—as will your budget and your tolerance for discomfort. I can't stress enough how important it is to make sure you go with a skilled doctor who has lots of experience and a good eye. Make no mistake, just as makeup is an art that requires trial and error to get it right, so are fillers and lasers. So choosing a doctor, in this case, becomes more than looking for a good medical technician, it is looking for an artistic eye and hand.

How do you identify a good dermatologist? Here are a few clues:

- Make sure the dermatologist is board-certified (check the American Academy of Dermatology: www.aad.org). This is a must and should be identified by the online presence of the doctor.

- Look for a dermatologist that practices primarily in the area of cosmetology; he or she will have much more experience than a general dermatologist. (The doctor's website should give you this information.)

- Arrange a consultation with the doctor and ask to see before-and-after photos of the procedure you are interested in pursuing.

- Get recommendations from friends who've had natural-looking procedures done.

I STARTED THIS chapter by saying that lipstick is the pushup bra of your makeup bag. There is nothing better to give your face a sexy boost than a great-looking lipstick that's been wisely chosen and well applied. Just like the Victoria's Secret catalogue says, there's "one for every moment and mood." But buyer beware in your quest for sexy smackers. Just as breast implants in the wrong hands can make your chest look like you are wearing water balloons, lip fillers can make you resemble a duck more than a duchess. Instead, read my lips: Your magic bullet is a creamy natural lipstick, outlined with an evenhanded lip liner, and carried with the confidence of a beautiful woman. (That would be you.)

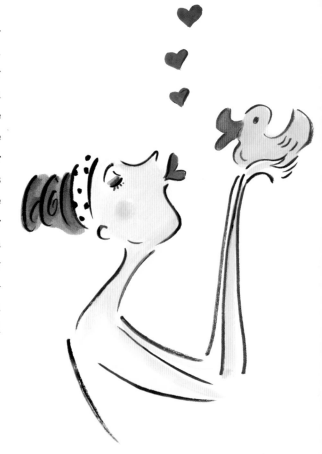

Some might consider lip brushes superfluous. Not so—just ask any good makeup artist. They have staying power worthy of investment. A mouthful of moist lipstick applied with a lip brush trumps the tube anytime for last and beauty—just try it. I love the Tom Ford Lip Brush #21 because it's taut enough to pick up a good amount of lip color from the tube but gentle on the lips and flexible enough to spread the color easily. That said, Tom Ford is a luxury beauty splurge, and you may want to try something less pricey. For that I suggest the following:

- Kevyn Aucoin Retractable Lip Brush—great for the purse and foolproof precision

- MAC #318 Lip Brush has lots of color pickup and is great for blending

- e.l.f. Studio Retractable Lip Brush

Here's a surprising ally in the quest for younger-looking lips: A good cosmetic dentist specializing in veneers.

Veneers can be contoured or built out to widen the lip's arch and increase lip support, resulting in a permanently plumped-up looking mouth. But like most cosmetic procedures, it is a pricey remedy: Veneers can cost up to $1,500 per tooth!

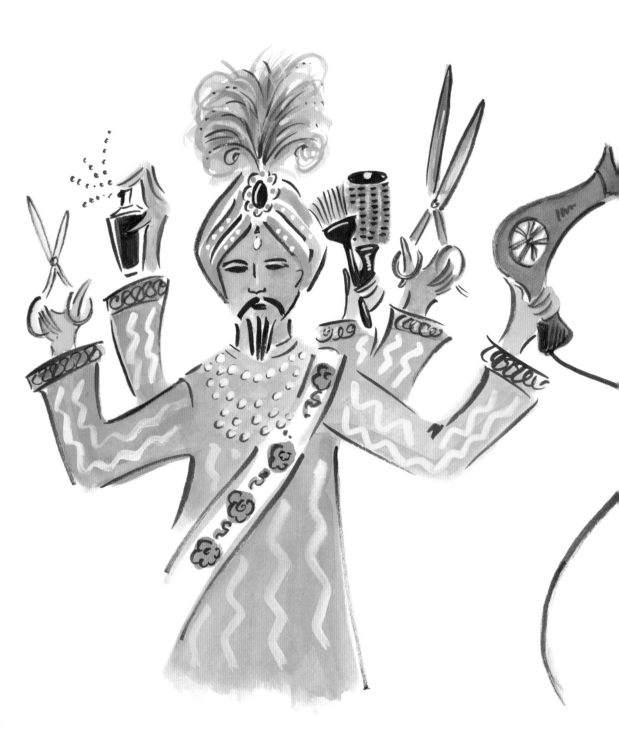

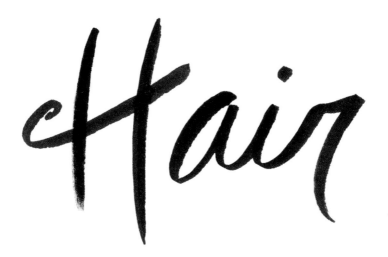

CHAPTER TEN

Hair

hair dos and hair don'ts

FIRST THINGS FIRST: ALL HAIR, YOURS AND MINE INCLUDED, SHOULD LOOK EFFORTLESS. YOU DON'T WANT YOUR HAIR TO BE SO OVER THE TOP THAT IT LOOKS LIKE IT'S HEADED TO A RED-CARPET RENDEZVOUS WITHOUT YOU.

At our age, casual, natural elegance is what we're going for—not helmet heads, shoe-polish mops, frosted frizzies, teased tresses, or highlight ODs. If you recognize your own hair in this paragraph, you may need a good hair guru to come between you and your current coiffure.

The truth is, unlike lipstick or eye-liner, hair is the only cosmetic you can't simply wipe off, so isn't it worth getting it right? Because getting it wrong can be a major beauty disaster. You can throw out an impulse purchase, or wipe off a frosted lipstick, but you can't just shampoo a cure into a bad coif—a few wrong moves with the scissors and you've got shear disaster. A cut too layered, too short, or too long can exaggerate the lines in your face and make your whole body seem out of proportion. And the wrong color can give you the Morticia Addams look, aging you instantly.

The truth is, unlike lipstick or eyeliner, hair is the only cosmetic you can't simply wipe off, so isn't it worth getting it right?

When it comes to women of a certain age, there are so many bad hair dos, and even more hair don'ts, that it's easy to get confused. For instance, you probably recognize some of these "rules" about hairstyles after fifty:

- "You shouldn't wear long hair."

- "You shouldn't wear bangs."

- "Get rid of the dark hair."

- "Add blond highlights to cover the gray strands."

But I don't believe in those rules, and neither do the famous hair masters I consulted. Take, for example, hairdresser Gad Cohen, who knows everything about haircuts and makeup (see www.gadcohen.com). He's styled great beauties from Jaclyn Smith to Jane Seymour. Or Louis Licari, Manhattan's go-to color genius and *Today Show* regular. (I've seen Ellen Barkin and Susan Sarandon in his Fifth Avenue habitat.)

Louis says, "The most common faux pas I see is when a woman says, 'I am this number of years old, so now I have to have lighter hair.'" And Gad says: "When you have good quality hair and the silhouette is right, you can have any kind of hair—including long hair. The right haircut is better than the scalpel."

Louis adds, "Hair is the best kind of makeup for the face." The right shade can enhance skin tone, complement a well-composed cosmetic palate, and, yes, even make you look more youthful.

This chapter will focus on how to determine the right cut and color that works best for you, and how to work with your hairdresser and colorist to help them make you look like yourself, only better.

I will also shed some guiding light on how to determine the right length for your hair, how to achieve the most realistic color, and when you can get away with doing color at home. And while I'm at it, I'll also explain why you should never cross your legs at the beauty salon, along with why lace is good for thinning hair. First, let's start with an important . . .

BEAUTY TRUTH:

Don't try to replicate the head of hair you were born with. You've grown up. So has your hair.

Don't look back! Don't attempt to freeze-frame the cut or color of your past. After years of time and sun exposure, your skin color has changed. That means your hair must change, too, in order to complement your face. As our faces morph, so must our hair.

But where do you look for inspiration? Certainly, models and celebrities have been setting hairstyle trends for decades. Remember Julie Christie's bob, Mia Farrow's pixie cut, Diana Ross's afro, and Farrah Faucet's feathered layers—not to mention Jennifer Aniston's "Rachel,"

which remains the most requested cut in history? But be forewarned: What you see isn't always what you get. Often, the pumped-up tresses you see on models and actresses in fashion magazines are not altogether real. I speak from experience when I tell you that many of those women are wearing wigs, hairpieces, hair extensions, or some combination of the above.

Case in point: I once had a photo shoot with a major pop music diva. Her iconic beauty look had a lot to do with her very large and thick head of hair, so of course we had brought along one of the best and most celebrated hairdressers in the world to work with her. But she declined his services, explaining that she worked exclusively with one hair artist who arrived glued to her hip, along with a huge suitcase of unknown contents.

"Hair is the best kind of makeup for the face."

Our hairdresser could not have been more gracious. He expressed his regrets about having missed the opportunity to work with the celebrity, and she seemed genuinely remorseful. But those of us who watched her getting ready for the camera learned that under that thick crown of hair and in that hairdresser's suitcase, a big dark secret lurked: She was almost bald! Her signature tresses, the ones that inspired a huge amount of hair envy and imitation and defined her physical presence, were in fact a series of wigs and hairpieces! When I saw her without the fakes, it took my breath away. That, of course, was why the chanteuse wanted no one except her own hairdresser—more accurately, her own wig master—within blow-dry distance.

Get a color that complements your skin tone, a cut that complements your body type, and don't get obsessed with what you can't have.

The lesson here? Don't be influenced by trumped-up celebrity styles. Find your own style that works with the hair you have, not the seemingly voluminous hair you see on celebrities of a certain age, because we now know that much of the time their

hair isn't real. Get a color that complements your skin tone, a cut that complements your body type, and don't get obsessed with what you can't have—especially since a quick glimpse in the mirror should prove you've likely got plenty to work with. Let's start with the essentials.

it's all about the cut

Here's the truth: A good haircut cannot—and should not—be underestimated. Back in the day (let's say the '50s and '60s) when hair salons were called "beauty parlors," you got a "hairdo." Your "beautician" set your hair in pincurls or rollers, put you under a dryer, and then "teased your hair" and "combed you out." An asphyxiating application of ozone-destroying hairspray was usually involved. Young women spent a lot of time worrying how they'd manage to look good after they got married. No, they weren't worried about "letting themselves go," they were trying to figure out how they'd manage their hair if they couldn't climb into bed each night with a helmet of pink rollers.

Enter the swinging '60s, when Vidal Sassoon changed the world with a pair of scissors. Though there aren't many people still

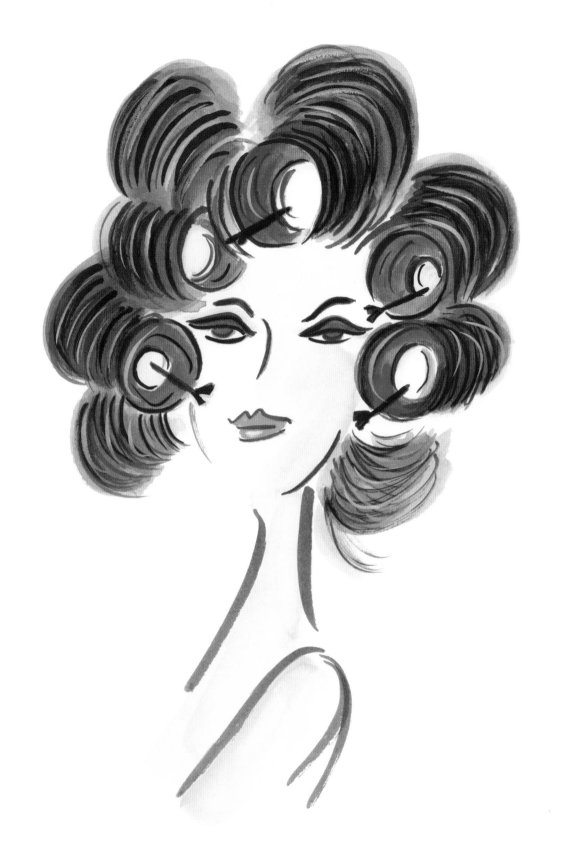

sporting the geometric cut he made famous, we're all benefitting from his revolutionary notion of ready-to-wear hair that required no rollers, hairdryers, or hairspray—but this assumes a lot of skill from the person doing the cutting.

"Length and volume should be dictated by your height and your weight—your shape."

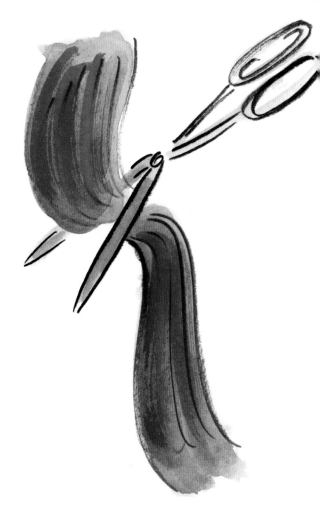

Here's the trick to getting a good haircut: proportion and balance. Hair should relate to the silhouette of your body. Gad says, "Length and volume should be dictated by your height and your weight—your shape."

His general rule of thumb: The larger and taller the body, the bigger the hair can be. If you're lean, your hair most likely will benefit from being the same: sleek and close to the head. If you're curvy, as a general rule, you need longer, fuller hair so your head doesn't look too small in contrast to your body. If you're shorter, you'll want a cut that gives height at the crown. The whole image must be taken into account, including your natural neckline and jewelry choices. For example, if you have a short neck, wear minimal jewelry. Keep earrings and necklaces simple and small and avoid big collars on blouses, sweaters and coats. Hair should be layered gently around your face.

Most women over fifty look best if they choose a length somewhere between the chin and just grazing the shoulder, with a cut that adds volume. And Gad says, "Use bangs instead of Botox." He suggests hair looks best at this stage of life with soft, imperceptible layers that are cut on the bias—that is, not in choppy layers, which are too artificial looking, unflattering, and dated.

Black women have a unique elasticity to their hair, which can be styled and worn close and cropped tightly to the head or stretched out for a longer look. Gad uses the shape of the head to determine the shape of the cut. Michelle Obama and Oprah Winfrey both wear longer hair that's been chemically relaxed, to great effect. As an alternative to that look and length, pull the hair back with a band and allow the hair behind it—on the crown and sides—to go unrelaxed and free. "That's a modern, totally empowering look," that Gad says is "wearing your essence." And if it works with the overall silhouette, shorter hair can look great on black women because they often have beautifully shaped heads and wrinkle-free skin.

the basics of color

"The main purpose of hair color is to complement and give contrast to your skin color so your facial features will come alive and you look fresh, younger, and vital," Louis Licari says. "If you have to wear more makeup to make a new hair color look right, you picked the wrong color."

So how do you get the right color if you're doing it at home? Louis says that all the big-brand, at-home DIY products are pretty good. What really matters is the shade you pick. And he warns, be careful. "Hair color is a bit like drugs. It's easy to become addicted, and a little goes a long way."

One great side benefit of using color on your hair is that it looks thicker. Individual hairs are covered with microscopic scales, like fish scales, and when you dye or bleach the hair, the scales open and never lay flat as they did before the chemicals were applied. Opened hair cuticles can become three times their usual size, but you will sacrifice shine and smoothness.

CHECK OUT THESE BRANDS FOR HAIR COLOR BEST BETS:

- Clairol Natural Instincts
- Clairol Nice 'N Easy Root Touch-Up
- Garnier Nutrisse Nourishing Color Crème
- L'Oreal Paris Excellence Creme

When it comes to making your color choice, the hardest person to get a good, objective opinion from is the one with the most at stake: you. Most of us view ourselves through a mental scrim that does for us what Vaseline or gauze on the camera lens did for movie stars back in the day—everything looks a bit blurry and not quite in focus: better, kinder, but not very precise and true. That's where smartphones come in. The pictures you can take on a cell phone are not always flattering (they don't call them kindphones), but you can really see what's right or wrong. So be brave! Click and delete later.

Asking a trusted friend for advice is also helpful, but only if you know she's going to be completely frank with you. (This is a much bigger decision than what color to paint the living room walls. Not everyone gets to see your living room.) Better yet, leave it to a professional whose aesthetic you trust. In the world of beauty salons, word of mouth can't be beat. Ask friends, acquaintances, or coworkers whose hair you admire for the name of the person who colors her hair. Admittedly, sometimes it's a bit tricky to ask someone you're not close to for this information, so resort to stealth compliments, and perhaps they'll fess up.

For salons in your vicinity, you can also refer to Yelp.com for business reviews from real customers. Often, stylists within these salons will be lauded (or criticized) for their area of expertise. You'll discover quickly whether there's a color connoisseur in your neighborhood or a shade charlatan leaving a trail of brassy tresses in his wake. As with any big change you embark upon—whether it's finding a painter for your living room or a colorist for your hair—always get a consultation and estimate before making a color commitment. Most experienced stylists will certainly accommodate your request to get an initial (free) consultation before you schedule an appointment with them. If not, take this as a bad sign! Short of that consultation, here are some color tips from Louis, based on skin tone, worth heeding:

VERY FAIR SKIN

Just about any color looks good unless you go to extremes. It's best to avoid deep browns and black (remember Morticia?). You want to avoid that witchy look. Also, pale skin is prone to ruddiness, and dark hair will only draw attention to redness in your undertones. Instead, choose blond, strawberry blond, and light brunette.

RUDDY SKIN

Avoid bright, red hair color; however, auburn would be a good choice, along with medium brown and golden brown.

CREAMY SKIN

Choose medium red tones, along with light browns and golden blonds. Avoid the harshness of dark browns and blacks.

MEDIUM TO OLIVE SKIN

Deep shades like mahogany will warm up your skin tone, but it's best to avoid red or copper tones, which can make your skin look sallow or orange—and avoid becoming blond. Make your hair too light and it can look like gray hair and drain color from your skin. Make it too dark and it can become monochromatic and shout, "I'm a wig."

DARK OR BLACK SKIN

At one time, African-American women thought their only color option was a semipermanent color to cover the gray, adding a tinge of red or going darker. "I think once hairpieces, extensions, and weaves became popular, Black women found a lot of other possibilities and became very creative with their hair, and they certainly started thinking in terms of different colors," Louis says.

And like fair skin, it works with a large range of colors. If you have golden undertones in your skin, try weaving caramel or cinnamon highlights around your face and through the ends, where the sun would hit. If you are more adventurous, you can even go blond (check out Rihanna in one of her hair color transformations, or Beyonce's blondish hues). Take care when mixing color with other chemical products like relaxants, and be aware that Black hair absorbs color much more quickly than Caucasian hair.

No matter what color your skin is, if you'd like to avoid the saturated, monochrome shoe-polish look that a bad dye job can bring, select a translucent color—not like an opaque paint, but rather more like a varnish, where each hair takes on a different tone. Louis says, "Tell your colorist, 'I'm a brunette. I'm happy as a brunette. But I don't want to look harsh. I want to see nuances in my hair. I would like to have most of my gray hair covered, but, if a strand or two shows through, that's all right.'" He explains, "This approach helps ensure your hair won't be too dark—and if it's too light, the colorist can always add color."

If you want a variegated look, you can put in highlights. But if there is too much contrast between the dark hair and the highlights, you'll look like an old-fashioned "frosty," which will make you look older and tacky. "Highlights shouldn't be too perfect or too bold," Louis says. "Perfect is imperfection." (Remember what I said in Chapter 2, about the concept of *Wabi-Sabi?* If not, reread.) What you're going for is a random collection of color, a thin stroke here, and a thicker stroke there that mimics what nature does.

Next to picking the wrong color, the second biggest hair color error, says Louis, is this: "Hairstylists think they have to work color from the roots to ends every time. But when you get a touch-up," he says, "get color on the roots only." And only work the color through to the ends for the last few minutes before taking it off. He recommends that everyone's hair should go from darker on top to lighter at the bottom.

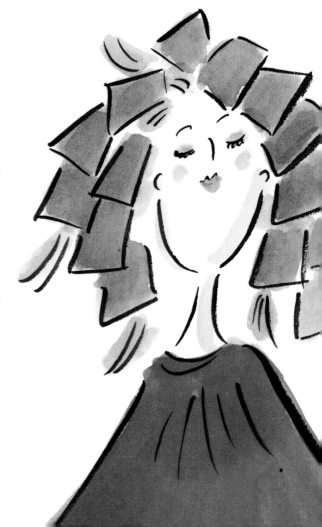

between appointments

In between salon visits, to cover up those gray hairs that sprout near your face and at your part (where they can make you look as if your hair is thinning), ask the salon to give you a formula to do minor touch-ups at home, or to give to the local salon in your winter or summer community. Don't be shy. Louis says he does it all the time to accommodate his customers when they are going away for extended periods of time and can't get in for a touch-up.

Also, friend and colleague formerly from L'Oreal, Joan Lasker, invented a brilliant product for gray roots between salon visits or DIY hair-color sessions called TouchBack. It is temporary hair color in a mistake-proof marker that bonds to the hair and holds its color until shampooed out, and it's available in eight shades.

This product was born out of Joan's personal need to cover the gray roots of her own beautiful hair. Joan had a fabulous career in the beauty industry and reinvented her professional self after fifty by starting her own business out of her house after her son went off to college. **Best Bets:** Women across the country have tried TouchBack (touchbackgray.com) and love it. And the product has been the recipient of Allure's Best of Beauty Award three times. Clairol Nice 'N Easy Root Touch-Up comes in a variety of shades as does Rita Hazan Root Concealer, and both work well for those times between.

DIY color

Thanks to the do-it-yourself trend of at-home products that imitate salon procedures, coloring has hit a high note in popularity. Advertisements make it look so effortless and easy. Who wouldn't want shiny, swishy hair like Andie MacDowell and Eva Longoria? For a fraction of a salon fee, a box of hair color is a steal and can deliver great results—but lest you want to end up with orange highlights or green hair, you MUST know what you are doing. If you're ready to color your hair at home, don't start before reading these simple rules.

1 BE CONSERVATIVE

It's best to go only a couple of shades lighter or darker than your natural color.

2 TRY BEFORE YOU DYE

Do a strand test before committing to the entire box. If the color turns out to be a bust, you only wasted $12. That's a bummer, but it's nothing compared to the hundreds you'd have to fork over to get it color-corrected by a professional! (See OOOPS! section later in the chapter.)

3 CHOOSE THE RIGHT SHADE

The color you see on the pack isn't going to look like the same shade on your head. A color expert once shared with me that if the hair color on the package picks up the pink or gold in your skin, then it's a shade that will suit you.

4 GO A SHADE LIGHTER

Select the ideal shade you are looking for, and then go a shade lighter because it's easier to go darker if you make a mistake than it is to make a dark shade lighter.

5 PREPARE YOUR HAIR

For color-staying power, be sure your hair is clean and well conditioned before you put color on it. It's best to wash your hair the night before you color.

6 ENLIST A FRIEND TO HELP

You don't want miss a spot on the back of your head.

7 CONDITION YOUR HAIR

After you rinse out the color, be sure to condition your hair, then do a deep-conditioning treatment at least once a week to preserve the color and nourish your hair.

Here's how to select the at-home color product that's right for you: It all depends on whether you're simply flirting with color changes, need gray coverage or a color boost, or you want something more permanent. Choose from those that wash out after a couple of shampoos to those that are permanent:

TEMPORARY COLORS
(LASTS 1–3 SHAMPOOS)

- What they will do: Add temporary color highlights and wash out quickly.

- What they won't do: Cover gray, lighten hair, or last very long.

SEMIPERMANENT
(LASTS 4–8 SHAMPOOS)

- What they will do: Can be used regularly to subtly enhance your natural color by adding a red tone to brown hair or a gold hue to blond, for example, or to disguise the first signs of gray. If you don't like the effect, these colors will eventually wash out.

- What they won't do: Lighten hair or give a dramatic, lasting color change or cover a high percentage of gray.

PERMANENT COLOR
(LASTS THROUGH 28 SHAMPOOS)

- What they will do: Give you a permanent color change—which means you'll need to touch up the roots every 4–6 weeks. Most will cover up to 100 percent gray (check the pack for details).

- What they won't do: It can't be washed out, period. If you make a mistake, visit a salon and hope for the best.

Once you have an idea of the level of color permanence you're looking for, you'll have to decide on what level of processing you want. Do you want all-over color or highlights? A quick pick-me-up, or a shine boost? Here are some facts to help guide you:

SINGLE PROCESS

A new color or toner is applied all over to create a new base color. The hair color is lightened and a new color is added in one easy step.

DOUBLE PROCESS

Typically used when lightening hair by more than two shades. First the hair is bleached to remove natural or colored hair pigments, and then pigment is added into the hair to create the desired shade. Since color is adjusted more than two or three shades, it's best to leave this process to the professionals.

HIGHLIGHTS

Adding highlights gives you more visible contrast than a regular single-process dye. Remember, less is more, and a few strands framing your face can offer you just the right amount of light to give skin a healthy glow.

GLAZES AND COLOR-ENHANCING SHAMPOOS

Use glazes, including tint formulas and color-enhancing shampoos, to help intensify a fading shade between salon visits. They revitalize color, smooth the cuticle, and add vibrant shine. To reduce hair damage, look for products that are ammonia-free. John Frieda offers a good selection, including Glaze Luminous Color, Glaze Clear Shine Gloss, Brilliant Brunette, Sheer Blonde, and Radiant Red, so one's bound to work for you.

Don't forget to wear something old when coloring your hair (if it stains your hair, it will certainly stain your silks, cottons, and polyester blends!), and smooth Vaseline along your hairline, on your ears, and on the back of your neck to create a barrier to keep dye from staining your skin.

OOOPS!

When hair color goes bad, I highly recommend you visit your salon for a quick fix rather than concoct another mixture to mess up your hair color even more. Remember, just dyeing over a color that might have gone too dark isn't a quick fix. Color cannot lift color. What does that mean? You can't remove black hair dye with light brown, blond, or any other lighter shade of hair color. You need special products to remove the color from your hair before it can be recolored. Purchasing other colors is a simple waste of time. There are products like Color Corrector by Salon Care Professional, which is a gentle, nonbleach blend of chemicals that oxidize permanent dyes. The kit comes with two, one-fluid-ounce bottles of product, which cannot be mixed until they are ready to be used. You choose your option according to your need. But again, I stress and recommend you visit a professional for best results. If you have any concerns, many at-home brands offer hotline numbers with consultants on call to answer any questions or problems (Clairol 1-800-CLAIROL and L'Oreal, 1-800-361-7358) are two of the most popular ones.

gray's anatomy

As for going totally gray: I think it can be dazzling on the right person, like my beautiful friend and colleague Jade Hobson, who is a former *Vogue* editor. But it only works if you have a complexion that has color and depth. It's best for someone with a slightly olive undertone and a lot of style. But you still have to take care of gray hair with the proper maintenance, including regular cuts, nourishing conditioners, and the occasional hair mask. Gray hair tends to be drier and coarser than hair that has retained pigment. Clairol Lights Shimmer or Artec White Violet Color Shampoo are great at-home treatments that contain bluing tints to prevent that "avoid-at-all-costs" yellowing effect, which comes from overexposure to certain elements like the sun or chlorine. Purchase moisturizing shampoos and alternate these with the above-mentioned products. Get occasional deep conditioning treatments or glazes at your salon; this will add shine while toning the hair to keep the brassiness away. Gray hair left unattended will never measure up to the beautiful statement it can make about entering your middle years, and it really will make you look old. But do it right, and this can qualify as another "wear your essence" moment, and thank you, Gad, for that concept!

hair quality and texture

Here is one of life's little injustices: As we age, the only body part that seems to get thinner is our hair.

After menopause, you have only about three-quarters the amount of hair you had as a younger person. (Though a few of the missing strands may turn up on your chin. But that's another story.) So what's the solution, other than hats? The medical options (at least for now) are limited to Rogaine or hair transplants (both show good results), and I'm not convinced that any of the home remedies or alternative medicines work.

Simpler and less costly approaches are products containing hair fibers and powders. Hair fibers, like Super Million Hair Enhancement Fibres, can be sprinkled on to thinning hair and will help camouflage trouble spots. They are available in a wide array of hair colors and seamlessly blend in with your natural hair. Hair powders not only color the scalp to conceal thinning hair but also help boost fine hair at the root.

hairpieces

Another option is to have a hairpiece made. But don't let the word fool you: it's more hairnet than wig, with large holes for your own hair to be pulled through. Real or synthetic hair that matches yours is tied onto the hair netting in very thin layers so it does not look bulky or wiglike. Once placed strategically on your head (usually on the crown or bangs, where it is often needed most), it secures into place with a flat small clip. It can be made to cover the entire crown, or just partially, and it blends easily with bangs. This is especially effective for hair that is curly, but it also works for straight hair.

While some might scoff at the idea of a "wig," you'd be surprised by how many celebrities with thinning hair use similar products. According to Louis, the high-end solution for celebrities these days is something called a "lace" hairpiece. It's a custom-made and imperceptible bit of lightweight fabric that looks something like a veil. It blends seamlessly with the skin of the scalp and with hair (real or synthetic) that has been matched to the natural hair.

SOME BEST BETS WORTH TRYING:

- Bumble and Bumble Hair Powder
- Nexxus Youth Renewal Rejuvenating Dry Shampoo
- Pssssst Instant Dry Shampoo
- TRESemme FreshStart Dry Shampoo

If your retreating mane could use a little mending, check local listings for wigmakers and have a consultation done. Prices and options vary, depending on the retailer, hair quality, and size.

hair extensions

Another more long-lasting solution to thinning hair can be found in the world of hair extensions. You need longer hair (chin to shoulder length) to camouflage them, and, if your hair is too layered, they show, but done properly, they're very effective. The process is somewhat laborious, as the hair extensions must be glued, woven, braided, or wrapped into your own tresses a few strands at a time. A good extension "job" should last two to three months and can withstand frequent shampoos and blow-drying. But you need strong hair to maximize the life of the extensions, so heed this warning from personal experience: My hair is very fine, and, when I tried extensions, the weight of the hair and glue put too much stress on my strands, and I ended up with a bald spot. If you have fine hair, it's better to avoid this nightmare altogether and instead opt for imperceptible clip-on extensions, especially if you want the extra confidence booster of full glorious hair

for a special occasion. Many a red-carpet walker uses this subtle technique, and only her hairdresser knows.

One caution: Whether you're using extensions, hairnets, or lace hairpieces, these remedies are expensive ($300–$5,000, depending on the choice and whether hair is real or synthetic). Be prepared.

a primer on hair products

What if you're not interested in faux tresses, but you could use some help finessing the hair you have? The shelves are full of hair-care products that promise all manner of magic—some that deliver and some that don't. The selection can be overwhelming, but it's helpful to know that all of them are designed to serve just one of five purposes: to add volume, to add shine and smoothness, to enhance natural curls, to strengthen weak hair, and to prolong hair color. You might find that you have several hair issues to address at once. You may want to add volume to smooth hair or want to preserve color and strengthen hair. There are several good products that work like cross-trainers and cover many bases when it comes to hair needs.

FOR VOLUME

This category of products creates the illusion of thickness and is designed for people with fine, limp thin hair. The easiest way to get volume is to invest in a volumizing shampoo because it is the most familiar form of hair product and therefore the simplest to manage. A volumizing shampoo works by leaving out most of the ingredients in regular shampoos and conditioners that weigh hair down and by removing the excess debris from around the root, allowing the hair to flow freely and unencumbered by weighty ingredients, giving the illusion of more volume. Since these products often compromise shine, it can be replaced by rubbing a dot of argan oil between the palms of your hands and fingers and stroking it through your hair. Or choose a modern formula that uses botanical alcohols to add lift, take away dryness, and compensate with ingredients such as wheat proteins that soften and add texture and shine.

Other volumizing products come in mousse, gel, and spray forms. These work by depositing hair thickening agents, such as proteins, keratin, and polymers, which coat the strands, increase the strand diameter, and temporarily make the hair feel and look thicker. Sprays seem to be the newest form, which help lift the hair at the root for volume and texture. A word of caution: Use these products sparingly because they can have the opposite effect when applied too amply.

Try these **Best Bets:**
- Oribe Dry Texturizing Spray (oribe.com)
- Oribe Shampoo and Conditioner for Magnificent Volume (oribe.com)
- Pantene Expert Age Defy Collection (Thickening Treatment, Shampoo, Conditioner, and Masque)
- Phytovolume Actif Volumizing Spray (sephora.com)

FOR SLEEK, FRIZZ-FREE, SHINY HAIR

You need hydrating shampoos and conditioners that contain conditioning oils such as argan oil to even out the hair shaft and create a smooth cuticle surface to promote shine. Finish with a leave-in hair conditioner to make hair less frizzy and more manageable. The newest versions are very effective and lightweight, using natural oils or silicones that allow hair to breathe and prevent a greasy or oily look.

Best Bets:
- Argana Mon Tresor (gadcohen.com)

- Garnier Fructis Sleek and Shine Fortifying Shampoo and Conditioner, Sleek Finish 5-in-1 Serum Spray (at most drugstores)
- Living Proof No Frizz Leave in Conditioner (livingproof.com)
- Matrix Biolage Smoothproof Shampoo, Conditioner, Serum and Leave-In Cream

FOR SOFT, DEFINED CURLS

In the past, harsh gels were the only tool in the arsenal for hair that is tightly curled, making the curls look hard and crisp. Research into the unique structure of curly hair has shown that it can be very fine, yet needs super conditioning to calm down the frizz. In general, the new prescription for this hair type is gentle shampoos with low or no harsh surfactants, coupled with lightweight creamy conditioners or sprays that coat the hair, defining curls and locking them into place.

Best Bets for Curl "Girls":
- Bumble and Bumble Curl Conscious Smoothing Shampoo and Conditioner (bumbleandbumble.com)
- Devachan DevaCurl Low-Poo Cleanser, One Condition and DevaCurl Set It Free Spray (devachan.com)

- John Freida Frizz-Ease Dream Curls Curl Perfecting Spray (at most drugstores)
- Motions Natural Textures Define My Curls Crème (at most drugstores—a fave for ethnic hair)

FOR STRONG RESILIENT HAIR

One of the biggest signs of aging (giving our neck and hands competition) is our hair. Since our hair is dead protein, it cannot repair and renew itself. It gradually wears out from environmental factors like sun and wind, chemical treatments, heat styling, and plain old brushing and combing. Untended hair at a certain point can look dull, lifeless, and broken. The solution is serious deep moisturizing and conditioning with proteins like keratin or fatty acids, which have ceramides that coat the strands and bind to the cuticle, filling in the cracks to help prevent breakage. Here are a couple of my favorites for the look of strong, beautiful hair:

Best Bets:
- Kerastase Resistance Bain Force Architect, Ciment Anti-Usure, and Masque Force Architecte
- TRESemmé Platinum Strength Strengthening Shampoo, Conditioner, and Heat Spray (at most drugstores)

FOR COLOR-TREATED HAIR

Most of us do color our hair, and, if you are anything like me, I try to stretch out the time between visits to my hair-color guru, Louis Licari. What I've learned is that normal cleansing agents in shampoos can sometimes literally strip away color, so, if extending the life of your hair color is your biggest issue, the best shampoo to use is a sulfate-free formula that employs a different cleansing system that doesn't "chelate," or extract the hair color molecules from the hair shaft.

Two on my **Best Bets** list:
- L'Oreal Paris EverPure Sulfate-Free Color Care System (at most drugstores)
- Pureology Hydrate Shampoo and Conditioner for dry, overprocessed hair (ulta.com)

UV light can also fade hair, especially in the summer months, so try a treatment spray like Redken Color Extend Total Recharge (redken. com)

THERE'S A REASON when we came of age that the biggest thing on Broadway was called *HAIR*. We're the first generation to embrace our "shining, gleaming, streaming, flaxen-waxen" birthright, and the ones who first understood that ready-to-wear hair is chic-er and more modern than anything created with pink, plastic rollers. There's no reason to allow a few gray hairs to make us give up now, especially with so many advances in at-home coloring and styling products. There's also no shame in walking into a salon and telling them exactly what we want—we did it with our male bosses decades ago, so this part should be easy. And taking charge of our own beauty, including our hair, is truly the ultimate 'do.

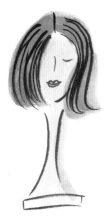
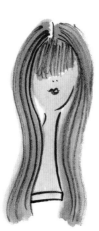
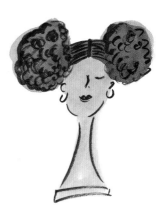

YOU SHOULD KNOW

According to famed hairdresser Gad Cohen, never cross your legs when you're getting your hair cut! Crossing your legs makes your spine shift, causing one side to be higher than the other. Instead, sit up straight and keep your shoulders even with one another.

When it comes to at-home hair color, some trusted brands have created new formulas that are healthier for your hair and easier to use. For instance, Clairol's permanent hair colors—like its Perfect 10 line—don't contain the ammonium hydroxide that's in most formulas. It smells a whole lot better and has a lower pH, which means it's gentler on the hair. Other formulations now also come in foam, making application much easier and less messy, thanks to its mousselike texture. Try John Frieda Precision Foam Colour for foolproof, drip-proof color. Another new advent in hair color is oil-powered color. Try Garnier's Olia line, which uses a blend of natural flower oils that improve hair health and shine, in addition to color.

Your hair isn't alive, but your scalp is! Treating your scalp like skin (which it is) can affect the look of your hair. Your scalp is aging just like every other part of your skin and probably experiencing excess dryness like you might have on other body parts and your face, due to the fact that cell turnover is slowing down. This can lead to a buildup of excess skin cell debris around the hair shaft and follicle, along with sweat and dirt, impeding the look of a healthy head of hair. If you treat your scalp like your face—with deep cleansing and moisturizing—you'll provide a smoother platform and environment for healthier-looking hair.

BEST BETS:

- Clear Scalp and Hair Beauty Therapy, Damage and Color Repair Conditioner
- Phyto Phytodensium Anti-Aging Shampoo

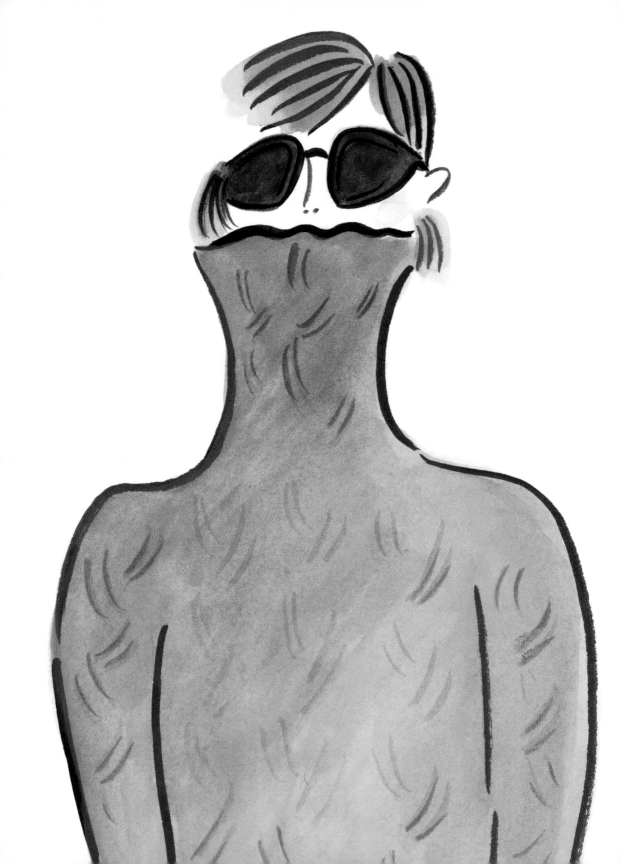

CHAPTER ELEVEN

THE FORGOTTEN ZONES

from the neck down to the hands up

I SPENT MOST OF MY ADULT LIFE WORRYING ABOUT MY BUTT AND BUST, NEVER ANTICIPATING THAT IN MY FIFTIES, MY ATTENTION WOULD BE DIVERTED TO ANOTHER BODY PART.

Alas, the moment arrived when I realized that the Thanksgiving turkey and I began to look like those "separated at birth" photos, and that my long, lean neck had to have been stolen by the body snatchers, who forgot to take my oversized butt at the same time.

The late Nora Ephron got this feeling completely, and that's why her book, *I Feel Bad About My Neck*, soared to the bestseller list. For many of us, this troubled drop zone, the increasingly declining curve between the neck and jaw that used to be a taut right angle, has made us feel, well . . . bad. Whether we wrap it in scarves, or hide it under a turtleneck sweater, many of us have become conscious of an area that only used to get attention during perfume application and jewelry shopping. Only a privileged few are granted an elegant, swan neck like

Only a privileged few are granted an elegant, swan neck like that of Audrey Hepburn— the rest of us fall into the "hide-the-slide" group.

that of Audrey Hepburn—the rest of us fall into the "hide-the-slide" group. Ephron was one of us, a reluctant participant, no doubt, in the acquisition of more scarves, chokers, and turtlenecks that accumulate steadily after one's fiftieth birthday. She nailed it when she said, "I often do what so many women my age do when stuck in front of a mirror: I gently pull the skin of my neck back and stare wistfully at a younger version of myself."

The neck is very delicate because, next to the eyelids, the skin in this area is some of the thinnest. As you age, it loses elasticity faster than anywhere else on your body, taking on the dreaded crêpe-y look. You should be every bit as diligent and careful about taking care of your neck and décolletage as you are about your face.

The same goes for your hands, which age just as quickly and require as much care and protection as our necks and chest.

The looming question: How do we prevent further "droppage" and bring back the illusion of a tight chin line, and how do we handle our fifty+ hands, now that gloves are no longer a "go-to" accessory? I wrote this chapter to answer these quandaries. You can start by heeding the following . . .

BEAUTY TRUTH:

It's okay to feel bad about your neck— and it's also okay to do something about it!

Let's discuss what you can do to prevent any real disasters from the chin down— without going under the knife.

neck neglect: what to do about it

We spend so much time and money trying to stave off the look of aging on our faces, but we often completely neglect our necks and chest. It's not until later, perhaps in our mid forties, that we begin to notice slight changes in the elasticity of the skin beneath our chins, or discover a growing tapestry of spots and lines on our once smooth and unmarked chests. By then, nature will have played some havoc with this delicate area, but the good news is that it is never too late to start damage control. If you don't already follow the basics of skin care from the neck down, begin NOW. Here's what you should be doing on a regular basis to help preserve—and refurbish—this sexy part of your body.

MOISTURIZE

Make sure you slather lotion or cream on your neck and chest every morning and night, and treat these areas to the same care you give your face. Moisturizers provide protection for the skin by limiting the evaporation of water from the epidermis, lubricating and softening its surface and therefore providing a comfortable and healthy appearance. Why deprive the neck of such nurturing?

EXFOLIATE

By getting rid of the surface cells and encouraging cell turnover, you will lessen sunspots and diminish the crêpe-y texture that suddenly seems to appear on your neck and chest. Specialty treatments like Retin A cream or glycolic peels work best but will only effect skin tightening, not the fatty skin lurking there. You should exfoliate once or twice weekly with gentle, nonirritating solutions and avoid grainy scrubs that can tear skin. Regular exfoliation equates with clean healthy glowing skin.

PROTECT

Slather on sunscreen. Like your face, the ultraviolet rays of the sun will take its toll on the elasticity of the skin on your neck if it's not protected. A sunscreen with an SPF of 15 is best and adequate since this will filter out about 93 percent of the skin-damaging UVB rays of the sun. This Sun Protection Factor will give you theoretically fifteen times the protection of your skin in the sun without any sunscreen. As mentioned in Chapter 3, anything over SPF 30 is a waste of money, since SPF 30 filters out 97 percent of UVB rays. Also consider wearing a brimmed hat when you're outdoors for long stretches—whether it's gardening, hiking, or lounging by the pool. The sun is strongest and most damaging between the hours of noon and 3:00 5* , but you should never leave the house without sunscreen, even if it's overcast. If you're active, be sure to reapply your sunscreen. Sweat will quickly wash the layer of sun protectant away, leaving your skin vulnerable to UVs.

Here are a few **Best Bets** for handling the basics:
- La Roche-Posay Anthelious 45 Body Ultra Light Sunscreen Fluid
- Lancôme Bienfait SPF 30 Lotion
- Olay Complete All Day Cream with Sunscreen, Broad Spectrum, SPF 15

Now that you have the preventative-care routine down, it's time to address the existing problems that have crept up over the last few years. See the common complaints below, and consider the cosmetic fixes before making the leap to lasers, fillers, and peels.

JOWLY CHIN LINE

A jowly chin line, the fatty tissue, or sagging area that begins to rear its droopy head on the lower jaw line, is most often noticed in its early stages in our forties and becomes progressively more noticeable during and after menopause. Jowls come from muscles slackening over time, and weight gain.

The Fix

Try using a color cosmetic to help camouflage jowls. Dark contouring powder or a darker foundation used under the chin creates the illusion of slimness and a tight jaw line. Or apply a self-tanner under the chin carefully along the jaw line and down the neck, continuing to the décolleté area for a longer-lasting effect.

Best Bets:

- Make Up For Ever Sculpting Kit
- Dior Bronze Self-Tanner Natural Glow Face

MOTTLED AND SPOTTY SKIN

Mottled skin is skin that has splotchy discolorations and age spots on the neck and chest. These patches and spots could be the result of changes in blood vessels, age spots due to overexposure to UVB rays, or hyper pigmentation (when the body produces too much melanin).

The Fix

Various methods can help mitigate this situation, including microdermabrasion, chemical peels, or laser therapy. This condition is best addressed by a dermatologist after the cause of the spots has been determined.

WRINKLY SKIN

At this stage of life, we all know what wrinkles are.

The Fix

I repeat, what works on your face should be used on your neck and chest, including sunscreens and those night products containing retinol, which over time can subtly help build collagen to improve elasticity and tone, reduce age spots, and smooth the skin. The most effective retinols, however, are prescribed by a dermatologist. Lasers have also been helpful by removing the top layer of skin and diminishing the surface wrinkles.

Best Bets:

- L'Oreal Skin Revitalift Anti-Wrinkle + Firming Night Cream
- Aveeno Positively Radiant Targeted Tone Corrector
- Your dermatologist

*we all know
what wrinkles are . . .*

For a more advanced turkey neck, the only effective tactic is to get yourself to a good dermatologist who knows how to use lasers, fillers at the jaw line, and Botox at the neckline where the chin meets the neck, to re-create that 90-degree angle. Botox will lift the sagging skin; filler (done in tiny doses along the jaw line) will improve the look of the chin line, and lasers will firm and tighten loose skin. It's not for everyone—and it's certainly not cheap—but if you look in the mirror and see that your chin and neck have formed a bigger merger than JPMorgan Chase, take action. Educated action, that is; make sure your dermatologist comes highly recommended and has thorough experience with injectables. (See Chapter 12 for detailed information about these and other cosmetic procedures and how they can help offset a host of other age-related skin issues.)

Now that we've figured out how to stop pulling our turtlenecks up, let's talk about how to stop pulling those sweater sleeves down and move on to the other telltale area of aging: our hands.

talk to the hand

You may wear sunscreen on your face every day, but does it make it on to your hands? Probably not, and then they suffer from sunspots and lines—and while we may feel at the top of our fifty+ game, our hands are suggesting otherwise. Prior generations turned to gloves to hide this spotty problem, but it's time to bring in the heavy artillery—not the lace and leather.

This section calls attention to your hands as an important part of your cosmetic routine. When hands are photographed in magazines, they look flawless, lineless, and veinless. Do you know why? Because the industry hires special hand models who will never touch a dish without a rubber glove, who will never expose their hands to the sun, who wear gloves most of the day, and who have their hands insured for gazillions of dollars. Right before the model's hands are photographed, the standard protocol is that she hold them above her heart for one minute. This trick reduces the amount of blood flow to the hands, making them appear smooth and perfect. These women are often not young like the fashion models seen in *Vogue* and *Vanity Fair*. They're generally in their thirties and forties, which illustrates how good hand care can keep your hands youthful forever. One hand model I know swears by almond oil

(Waleda Almond Soothing Facial Oil), which has high amounts of vitamins E and A. She's tested hundreds of creams and believes this inexpensive emollient penetrates the skin better than any hand cream. That said, many celebrities (as they move into their forties) swear by something else—Photoshop—to erase signs of aging from their hands that appear in magazine profiles, product endorsement ads, and movie posters. Fortunately, you don't need high-tech hijinx, just a few quality products and some common sense. Here are some other tips that make the most of our most-used extremities.

PAMPER YOUR CUTICLES

Keep your cuticle pusher in the shower, and, while your cuticles are warm and wet, push them gently back so they frame the nails. Avoid trimming, which only makes them look ragged if not done correctly. Apply an oil afterward (CND Essentials Solar Oil Nail & Cuticle Conditioner is a cult favorite and seems to work on the driest and roughest cuticles—which would accurately describe mine).

CUT AND SHAPE YOUR NAILS CONSERVATIVELY

Use an extra-fine emery board and file to a rounded shape. Forget square or pointy— shapes come and go, but the best nail shape to use is the classic curve. This gives you the most natural look. Added benefit: Rounded nails are less likely to break than square shapes. (And nothing looks worse than overly long, unkempt nails of various lengths. As for nail art, leave that to your daughter—along with lip gloss and texting "LOL" to your boyfriend.)

WEAR GLOVES WHILE WASHING DISHES

Madge was right, protect your hands. Chemicals and hot water can strip away the protective lipid barrier on your skin, making it susceptible to irritation and dryness. And remember to apply a layer of lotion to your hands each time you put on your rubber gloves—not only will it protect them, it'll give you an extra dose of moisture.

KEEP LOTION EVERYWHERE

Place a hand-cream pump at every sink in your house, on your bedside table, and stash travel-size tubes in your desk drawer and purse so you'll never forget to moisturize. Nivea Cream's travel-size tube is around a dollar and it's the perfect size for portability.

MOISTURIZE YOUR HANDS EVERY NIGHT

Always go to bed with a layer of moisture on your hands (Kiehl's Ultimate Strength Hand Salve and Jurlique Rose Hand Cream offer good dry hand relief), and/or use the excess on your hands after moisturizing your face. Every now and then, slather your hands in moisturizer and add cotton gloves to your night of sleep (yep, just like your grandmother did) for the added benefit of an at-home spa treatment.

KEEP YOUR HANDS AND NAILS MAINTAINED

Another must for youthful hands: Take them to the manicurist once a week. And BYOB—or shall I say, BYOP, for "Polish"—as many salons dilute their nail polish formulas. But who else is going to spend ten minutes giving you an amazing hand massage? The boyfriend? Well, maybe on the first few dates. The husband? I don't think so. And while you're there, pamper your toes and feet. They need some TLC any time of the year—no need to wait until sandal season.

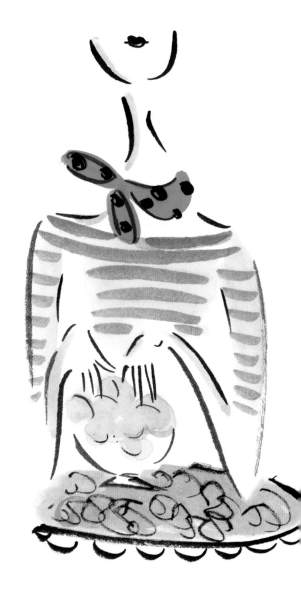

Of course, your nails are just as big a give-away as your skin. It's a rare fifty+ hand that can pull off a bright red, fuchsia, or orange polish. Darker skin allows for broader choices, but, if you fall into the fair-skinned category, bright colors will only emphasize veins and skin discolorations. Leave those fun colors to your toes. That said, it doesn't mean you can't "nail" a good color for your fingers. You just need to consider what works and what doesn't for your skin tone. Read on for the scoop on the nail-polish color spectrum, and what's right for you.

fingernail facts

Let's start with some inside dirt on fingernail polish: Did you know that most American brand name nail color is made in just two labs in the USA? Most large cosmetic companies, with the exception of Revlon, which makes its own, don't create their own nail color formulas. I recall attending a meeting at a nail laboratory, and being amazed at how many big cosmetic companies used this lab to fill their bottles and claim the formula as their own product. The nail polishes themselves are created by the nail lab—it's only the nail brush that each cosmetic company owns. Like with mascara, the brush is all important. Why? The brush

can add to the formula's performance in application, and many companies have patents to protect this asset—L'Oreal Paris and Sally Hansen, for instance, have some of the best brushes in the business. But don't

> Like with mascara, the brush is all important.

believe the hype when a label tries to justify outrageous prices with claims about longevity and chipping, especially since your favorite salon brands, like Essie and OPI, are owned by mass cosmetic companies (L'Oreal and Coty, respectively). So the next time you make a nail polish purchase, make it color-driven and price-worthy. No need to splurge on a Chanel polish. Save your money for a Chanel handbag instead, and try Essie nail color, which has a funny way of resembling the Chanel fashion shades we love so much.

But which "P" should you keep in your purse for manicure days? Finding the right nail polish for your skin tone can be as tricky as finding the ideal foundation shade. And choosing the right nude is harder than you think. Here are some tips to keep in mind while selecting color:

FAIR SKIN

This skin tone allows you to wear a bevy of colors, from light to medium. For barely-there shades, choose a clean, nude color, which counters any redness in your skin. Stick with pink or purple undertones for skin tones that are bluish white, and yellow undertones for skin tones that are creamier. Unless your hands are smooth and vein free, avoid anything bright or flashy, which will make your hands look old.

Best Bets:

- Essie Ballet Slippers
- L'Oreal Colour Riche Nail Polish in How Romantic

MEDIUM SKIN

Brighter shades will look better on you because vibrant shades enhance your skin tone and will make it appear tan or darker than it actually is. Brighter shades of pink, as well as orange with a warm neutral base, are your best choices. Avoid undertones that are too silvery or cool; they will clash with your warm skin tone. A good natural midtone nude to look at is Essie Nail Polish in Not Just a Pretty Face. But consider the following

Best Bets:

- CoverGirl Outlast Stay Brilliant Nail Gloss in Totally Tulip
- OPI Nail Lacquer in Tickle My France-y

DARK SKIN

Very dark skin looks fabulous with dark shades of polish. Deep plums, reds, and browns tend to look great when the hand is smooth and veinless (you can even get away with bright shades on smooth dark skin). The deeper your skin, the darker the nude should be. Avoid shades of white or very pale colors. Essie Nail Polish in Jazz offers good depth of color and is nude in undertone. For a little more neutral sizzle, try these:

Best Bets:

- L'Oreal Colour Riche Nail Polish in Greyt Expectations
- OPI Nail Lacquer in You Don't Know Jacques

When I worked at Revlon (where, as I mentioned, they *do* make their own nail polish), I had a male boss who was extremely insistent on my nails always being done (after all, it was Revlon!), and he noticed when they weren't. I'd walk into a big meeting, and, instead of focusing on my marketing plans, he'd say, "Andrea, nail color is one of the hallmarks of this company, and you have bare nails? Not acceptable." I've always worn clear polish, or natural if anything, but, while I had this job, I kept a stash of nail colors in my desk drawer. Before a big meeting, the nail polish fumes gave me away as they followed me down the corridor and into the boardroom. I was never very good at painting my own nails, and my desk looked more like a "Spin Art" station than an executive's workspace, with splattered lacquer and acetone remover stains everywhere. Once, I spilled an entire bottle of "Fire and Ice" on it, just as he was coming into my office—I was literally caught red-handed.

Don't follow my rushed example. Get a manicurist you trust, and visit her often. I always think that a good mani-pedi is better than a visit to the shrink. And though you should certainly pay the few extra bucks for a massage, my version of a "happy ending" is ten perfectly lacquered nails, and polished hands worthy of gesturing and flirting over the next seven days.

YOUR HANDS AND your neck can reveal telltale signs of age faster than a driver's license—but they can also continue to be hallmarks of your natural elegance and beauty. Leave the turkey necks for Thanksgiving dinner. Like Nora Ephron says, it's okay to feel bad about your neck

> Your hands and your neck can reveal telltale signs of age faster than a driver's license—but they can also continue to be hallmarks of your natural elegance and beauty.

and to worry about your hands, the good news is that you can do something about it. Just remember your VIPs (Very Important Parts) are still alluring and sexy, just like the rest of you.

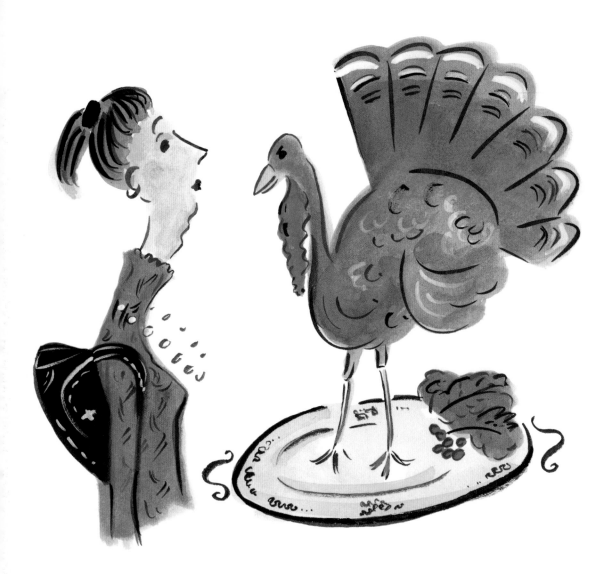

YOU SHOULD KNOW

If your neck has taken on the look of Tom Turkey, in all his wattled glory, consider liposuction. Dermatologist Dr. Gervais Gerstner, clinical professor of dermatology at Mount Sinai School of Medicine, recommends this procedure as an effective way of getting rid of a turkey neck, since it's caused by fatty deposits. And no amount of exercise or over the counter neck cream will remedy this. The procedure removes the fat buildup in your neck and under your jaw, producing great results for those afflicted with double chins. Sometimes, liposuction is combined with a laser procedure to simultaneously tighten skin.

Cost: Approximately $5,000.

Quick tip for hands: Don't forget to slather them in sunscreen when you're out and about, especially when you're on the go—literally. When you drive, your hands are vulnerable to sun damage, since they're exposed as they grip the wheel. If you're the "girl" in the convertible with the top down and your hair is blowing in the wind (and I hope you are), be doubly sure to dose your hands.

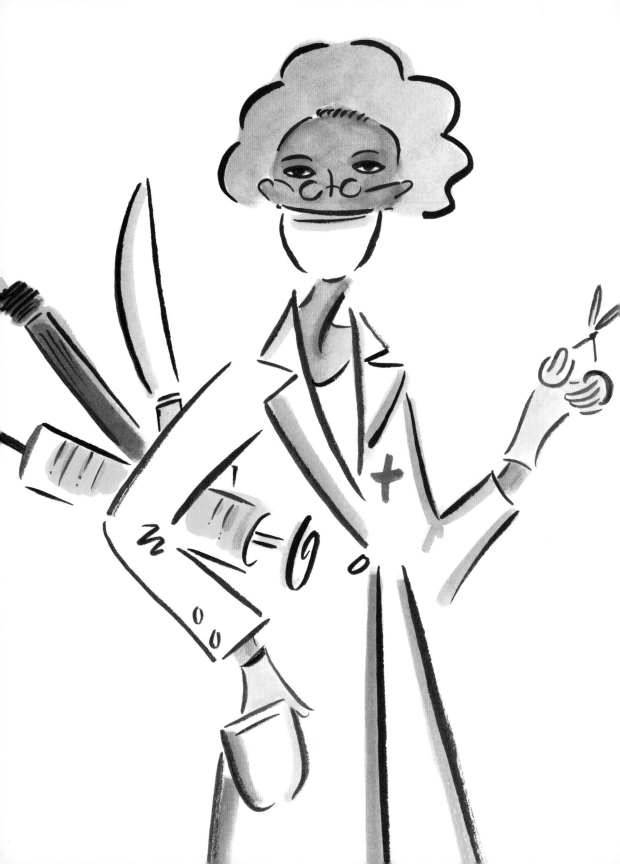

CHAPTER TWELVE

Cosmetic Tweaks

the needle, the knife, the know-how

LET'S BE FRANK: AT THIS POINT IN OUR LIVES IT IS SO VERY OKAY TO BE VAIN. IT TOOK ME YEARS OF PRACTICE, BUT HERE I AM, MRS. VAIN GLORIOUS, BEING KIND OF BOASTFUL ABOUT HOW I'VE LEARNED TO EMBRACE MY VANITY.

If you have, too—welcome to the club. If you haven't—no problem (and most likely, you're not reading this book, anyway).

There are women who've never missed a day of exercise, but rarely (or never) have worn makeup except to their child's wedding. I like to think I have a foot in both camps. Everyday exercise is something I try to accomplish, but I'll admit I still like getting asked about my minimal makeup or hair, or my toenail polish. The feminine ritual of maintaining my appearance makes me feel energetic, youthful, and together. And when others appreciate it, so much the better. It's a little like tending to a garden, weeding and cutting to make it bloom to its most beautiful best, or restoring parts of a house to give a platform to its natural elegance.

I certainly do want to look like myself, only better . . . not for him, not for them . . . for me.

I fully comprehend the fact that confidence and true beauty come from within, but I also embrace the notion that well-being can be enhanced by maintaining a look of health that exudes the energy of youth and vitality. And if you've learned one thing about me from reading this book, I certainly do want to look like myself, only better . . . not for him, not for them . . . for me.

We are, at this stage of our lives, in full control of how we present ourselves to the world. It's kind of fun to feel empowered enough to flip the middle finger at the toll that having a good long life has exacted on our looks. So here's my thought for you: If you believe in going through life looking as good as you can, and keenly feel you want to reclaim some of your physical beauty—stick with me on this one—it may mean using not just what you've learned here about makeup, but also investing in some capital improvements via more involved cosmetic enhancements. And by "enhancements," I mean anything from chemical peels to eye lifts. Taboo territory? *Uh uh*—not any longer.

Chances are, if you look around you, you'll see that "the face of change" is beginning to happen among your peers. Have you been to any thirty- or forty-year college reunions yet? I have. And chances are, a few of your friends have even had some kind of "work," whether it's Botox, lasers, fillers, or possibly the "hard stuff," by which I mean adjustments involving the scalpel—plastic surgery. And chances are, that number is higher than you think.

"Does she or doesn't she?"

Nowadays, it's a little like finding out who lost her virginity in high school. By the time we graduated, there were few who hadn't, and those who had were beginning to kiss and tell.

Perhaps you're realizing that using moisturizers, sun protection, and other skin solutions isn't doing enough to keep your face as fresh as you'd like, and you're now thinking, *Should I or shouldn't I?* If so, you're not alone. According to the American Society of Aesthetic Plastic Surgery, nearly 10 million procedures are done every year. And while 80 percent represent procedures such as Botox, lasers, and fillers, the other 20 percent are surgical (from liposuction to nose jobs).

Sure, in our twenties and thirties, we probably claimed we'd never use fillers, let alone undergo any form of plastic surgery. I certainly said, "Never ever!" But guess what? We've changed, and perhaps more important, so has the technology. The types of treatments available now didn't exist twenty years ago. They're less invasive, less uncomfortable, and more effective than ever. And while I will never be a proponent of face-swapping plastic surgery and over-the-top injections (sorry, Joan, you've gone too far),

I'm totally on board with taking advantage of cosmetic breakthroughs to spring out of the physical rut of age-related doldrums—with one caveat: Be conservative.

surface issues: lasers, fillers, and botox

If you're considering any of these cosmetic procedures, you want to find a good doctor, one who has a long history and rate of success with all of the procedures I am about to discuss. New York–based dermatologist Dr. Gervaise Gerstner (you met her in my chapters on lipstick and necks), who has refinished, refined, and reshaped countless faces, says the average age of her patients is forty-three, but it is skewing younger each year, with women in their twenties and thirties—along with a growing number of men—starting to form a sizable base in her practice as well. Below are some of her more commonly used procedures:

be conservative . . .

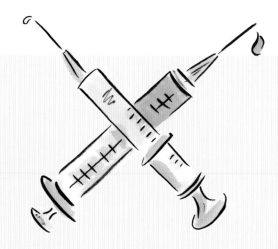

LASER TREATMENTS

Even those with advanced signs of aging can benefit from lasers, which resurface skin, diminishing wrinkles, scars, red spots, and sun damage. The goal of this procedure is to reveal healthy and even skin. Recovery time varies depending on the depth of the treatment. Some of Dr. Gerstner treatments include Lumenis Duet Hair Removal, Candela V Beam, and the lasers from Solta Fraxel Re:store Dual, Clear + Brilliant, and Thermage, which she uses for tightening of the neck.

- RISKS: Discomfort during procedure, temporary redness, skin flaking.
- COST: Approximately $350 to $2,000 per treatment, depending on the type of laser.

BOTOX

This injectable drug revolutionized the beauty industry. Botox is a bacteria called *Clostridium botulinum*, and, when used in small targeted doses, it helps to weaken and relax the nerve impulses, disengaging the muscles that give you that permanent furrow on your forehead, the vertical lines at the top of your nose, and other facial wrinkles. The desired result should make you appear softer and less wrinkled, less angry-looking (despite not feeling that way), and less

worried. And yes, more youthful. The effect lasts three to six months.

- RISKS: Too much Botox will give you a shiny forehead and a frozen, deer-in-the-headlights look (see most of the women from the *Real Housewives* franchise as a cautionary tale). In a small percentage of cases, there can be drooping of the eyelid (ptosis), headache, difficulty swallowing (when injected around the neck), dryness of mouth or eyes, and neck pain. And of course, discomfort at the injection site.
- COST: Approximately $400 to $800.

DERMAL FILLERS

Sometimes referred to as "liquid facelifts," these are procedures that offer some of the benefits of a surgical facelift without the long recovery time. Fillers like Restylane, Juvéderm, and

Belotero give you a youthful fullness, enhance shallow contours, and smooth away facial lines and wrinkles. I used Restylane regularly, which filled in and smoothed out my skin, especially the vertical folds that appear by the side of the nose, and the "puppet" lines around the mouth. It also helped stave off spending the big bucks on a neck lift . . . for a while, anyway. It lasts for six to nine months.

- RISKS: Localized pain or discomfort at injection site, redness, swelling, bruising (in some cases).
- COST: Approximately $600 to $1,000 per vial.

IPL (INTENSE PULSED LIGHT) TREATMENT

This procedure helps the appearance of sun-damaged skin by removing redness caused by broken capillaries, sunspots, freckles, and brown spots. IPL Treatment utilizes intense, broad-spectrum, pulsed light to help erase these particular issues with no downtime and great results within a short period of time. To see full results, it usually requires four or five treatments, depending on the issue. The effect is permanent, providing you stay out of the sun.

- RISKS: Temporary, mild swelling, redness, brown-spot crusting, occasional bruising, and superficial blisters.
- COST: Approximately $300 to $500 per treatment.

CHEMICAL PEELS

These procedures improve the texture and appearance of the skin by using a chemical solution that causes dead skin to slough and peel off, fostering cell renewal and collagen production. Chemical peels are great for addressing issues of aging (fine lines and even deeper wrinkles), acne, sun damage, and hyperpigmentation, and you'll see visible results after one procedure, depending on your particular issues and the chemicals used. Some mild peels that Dr. Gerstner uses are Salicylic, Glycolic, and Melange peels. The downtime involved is none to three weeks, depending on the peel.

- RISKS: Discomfort or pain, redness, swelling, scabbing and crusting, depending on the depth of the chemical peel.
- COST: Approximately $250 to $5,000, depending on the type of peel.

I'm a big proponent of safe and conservative (underscore safe and conservative) cosmetic tweaks for many reasons:

- The results last for several months (three to nine months, depending on where on the face/neck it is used).

- The changes can be dramatic yet not detectable.

- Some procedures can be done before work, after work, or at lunch time (the appointments never take more than an hour).

- There's no long recovery process.

However, fair warning: Any of the above "noninvasive" cosmetic procedures can be performed unwisely in the hands of the wrong doctor, so diligently check your doctor's expertise, and start with small tweaks until you are comfortable with the dermatologist's skill and handling of your face. Understand and know the slippery slope of dermatological fillers so you don't wind up like so many of those "freaky-faced" Hollywood celebrities—beware of big lips, frozen brows, a bulbous forehead, and over-plumped cheeks. Leave those exaggerated looks to Barbie dolls and reality TV stars.

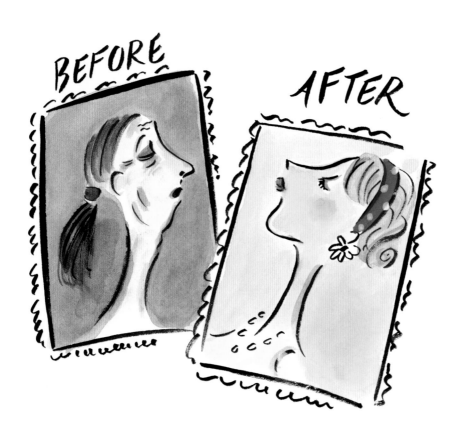

If you're considering visiting a dermatologist for any of these procedures, Dr. Gerstner recommends keeping in mind the following questions:

1 Is the dermatologist board certified?

2 How experienced is the doctor at using the technology/procedure you are considering?

3 Is the doctor interested in your general health (e.g., Does she/he do a melanoma check on first visit and annually after that)?

4 What is the doctor's aesthetic when it comes to fillers and Botox? (Gerstner suggests looking for answers like "less is more," "rested," "healthy," "natural," "soft," and avoid doctors who believe in the "California, celebrity, red carpet, or big cheek" look.)

5 Is the doctor listening to your needs, desires, and bothersome skin issues rather than telling you what you need (the latter comes with time and trust)?

6 Does your doctor discuss all options for treating your particular skin issues?

7 Does the doctor ask you about your history of sun exposure and whether you have a family history of skin cancer?

diligently check your doctor's expertise . . .

the last frontier

I have to admit, there was a time when Botox and fillers were a lunch-time (or after work) maintenance thing with me, on the same schedule as getting my hair highlighted—pretty much every three or four months. But cosmetic surgery required a lot more thought, angst, and, in my case, a good dose of Catholic guilt about spending a boatload of money on this narcissistic pursuit. Facing the reality of getting a face-

Facing the reality of getting a facelift reached deeply into the dark side of my vanity: Was this unmentionable procedure full of deceit?

lift reached deeply into the dark side of my vanity: Was this unmentionable procedure full of deceit? Did it cross the line into my fears about aging and touch the underbelly of my lost youth? Was I in denial and didn't want to acknowledge it? Was I surrendering my notions about aging gracefully? I do know it treaded somehow uncomfortably on the frank territory that overlaps cosmetic products, which I use and believe in, and was perfectly happy to discuss, guilt-free.

When I finally made an appointment with a plastic surgeon, I was hoping the doctor would send me away with, "You don't really need my services." No such luck . . .

A good friend admitted to me that she had a facelift, so she was some help, but her face—which looked great—was not my face. Also, it didn't help that my imagination took flight with all the things that could go wrong. In the spirit of spilling it all, when it got to the point where I couldn't stand my neck anymore (and my dermatologist couldn't stand to hear my complaints any longer), I contacted Dr. Rosenberg, a New York City facial plastic surgeon who is part magician, part artist, part shrink. He talked me through all my fears and questions—I mean, can you imagine having me for a patient?

His brilliant hands have recrafted the face of many people, from politicians to movie stars to women like you and me. I kept telling myself it was only an informational meeting, because I was very nervous. I mean, God forbid something should happen to me on the operating table—what would my kids say when they learned how I'd met my final end? "Rest in peace, Mrs. Robinson. She died trying to get her neck back." No thank you!

Dr. R. got my anguish on this one immediately, and said, "Mrs. Robinson, you're afraid you won't wake up, right? I have never lost a patient and I assure you, you will not be the first." Suddenly, with that simple reassurance addressing the top of my fear list, I felt calmer. Ultimately I made the decision to move forward with the procedure. I'm not minimizing that it was costly and uncomfortable—recovery took about seven days in my case. But think of it this way: IT'S YOUR FACE! It's more expensive to buy a car than to fix your face—and you don't guzzle gas money, require collision insurance, or need a monthly parking space.

Here, some wise observations from Dr. Rosenberg that may ring familiar to those of you considering plastic surgery (even if it's only in secret, in your head). He says, "When women reach an age (usually in their late forties or early fifties) where, typically, their hormones start diminishing, they rapidly notice a change in their facial structure, and, over a very short period of time, they stop recognizing themselves in the mirror. So this vibrant, often fit person who is taking care of herself looks in the mirror, and, despite all her work, she sees a tired face. That starts to affect how she feels about herself . . . no matter how hard a woman works out, and how well she eats, the face ages at a certain point. There is often a dissatisfaction and a disconnect—'who is this person in the mirror?' And that starts to lead to a sense of loss—a loss of who they were physically."

He adds, "What makes people happy after surgery is that they've regained something, and they are able to extend that period in their lives where they feel vibrant and attractive. So there's a sense of well-being that comes from taking care of themselves, and seeing how well they can look again."

> But think of it this way: IT'S YOUR FACE! It's more expensive to buy a car than to fix your face—and you don't guzzle gas money, require collision insurance, or need a monthly parking space.

His philosophy? "Youth is not the magic potion. What I'm trying to do is not necessarily make people look younger; I'm trying to make them look beautiful now. So that when they look in the mirror and see a reflection, it feels familiar, and they feel excited about what they see, and comfortable in their own skin" (if you've been following this book's ultimate message of "Look like yourself, only better," you'll recognize this sentiment!).

Don't be afraid to explore plastic surgery when considering your options; it's only a consultation, and the information you will acquire will make a huge difference in how you feel about proceeding—or not.

Dr. Rosenberg describes his consultation methods this way: "I always begin the same way, by asking a patient how I can help her. I hand them a mirror and ask her to identify what bothers her. It's a very big decision to think about having elective surgery, so I listen carefully and very quickly can assess how much surgery the patient can handle.

Most often, this opens a door, and she will ask me what I pick up on, and we 'walk through' her face together. I always underscore that the goal is to make her look as good as possible without a sign of surgery."

There is a case to be made for plastic surgery. It's not for everyone, but it may be for you. Don't be afraid to explore it when considering your options; it's only a consultation, and the information you will acquire will make a huge difference in how you feel about proceeding—or not. The consultation cost is most often deducted from the final bill when moving forward with the procedure, but I recommend getting two so you can compare physicians and approaches. And when you do, be sure to follow this . . .

BEAUTY TRUTH:

Cosmetic surgery is an acceptable option— just be smart about why, when, where, and with whom to choose it.

it's not for everyone . . .

Here are some questions you should always ask your doctor before committing to a plastic surgery procedure.

1 How many procedures like mine have you performed?

2 Can you show me before-and-after photos?

3 What are the risks associated with this procedure?

4 Are there alternative treatments for my issues?

5 What is the recovery like?

6 When will I begin to see results?

7 Where will you perform the surgery?

8 Is there anything that you recommend I do or take before the procedure to ensure better results or a quicker recovery?

9 What type of anesthesia will you use?

10 What complications could occur?

11 Are you board certified?

12 What is the total fee, including you, your anesthesiologist, cost of the operating room, and any other assistance required?

And here are some questions that Dr. Rosenberg says you should ask yourself while meeting these doctors:

1 Is the place clean? Assess the atmosphere of the office.

2 Is the staff respectful and discreet?

3 Is there attention to detail? Is it a quiet, low-key, well-maintained environment?

He comments further, "Everything matters. This is about detail. To do surgery on someone, and do it well, you need to be a detail-oriented person. If you don't see an office that's run well, then you have to question the person who will be touching you—how will he or she run his operating room?"

know thyself

True, a few injections can iron out forehead creases and deliver plump cheeks. And while it's safe to assume that furrowed brows will never be in vogue, other issues like jowls and necks can require the scalpel, so choose treatments wisely—and sparingly.

If your motive is to trade in your physical identity for someone else—and if you think looking flawless means any actual flaws in your life will melt away after the surgery—you aren't being fair to yourself.

It's not about seeking perfection, it's about feeling better about yourself—the *Wabi-Sabi* way. And yes, while Angelina Jolie may be beautiful, she hasn't raised your kids or conquered your office issues, so forget about who's on the *Vanity Fair* cover and just do you because you are the best thing about YOU. Recognize that cosmetic surgery is an imperfect art—or, as Dr. Rosenberg puts it, "an individual surgeon performing a craft, working on a person's face within its limitations. The surgeon can only work with what he is given."

WHEN DONE FOR the right reasons and with a skillful surgeon, the results of a cosmetic procedure will be really satisfying. And the beauty of it all is that we can remain attractive at any age, whether it's from good genes, good decisions, good makeup or—when appropriate—good doctors.

we can remain attractive at any age . . .

YOU SHOULD KNOW

Here are a few tips from dermatologist Dr. Gervaise Gerstner about cosmetic enhancements and daily maintenance for treated skin:

If you're considering fillers (such as Restylane, or Juvéderm), she feels two vials of filler, max, should be used per visit.

If you're looking into peels, she favors glycolic peels over traditional facials (for value and results), and believes that the following three rituals help keep skin looking its best:

- Sunscreen daily

- Glycolic peel pads used three times a week

- Retin A (pea-size dose) once a week

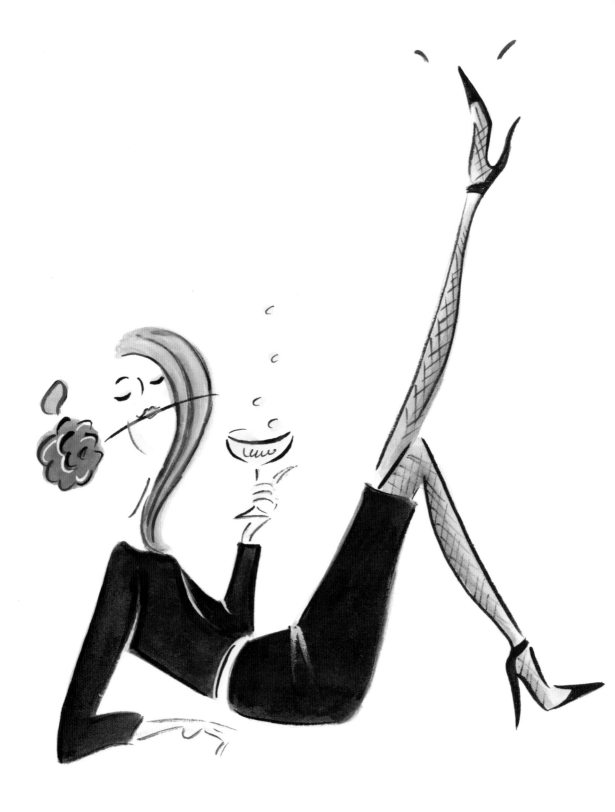

Sexy Doesn't Have an Age

I HAVE TO ADMIT IT . . . I LOOK FORWARD TO WATCHING THE GOLDEN GLOBES AND THE OSCARS TO SEE WHAT THE SCREEN GODDESSES ARE WEARING, AND EACH TIME I ADMIRE THE SMALL MIRACLES IN CELEBRITY MAKE OVERS.

I am always inspired—yes, inspired—when Janet has lost weight or Ellen's gotten a new haircut or Julianne has tried new eye makeup because it moves me to think about self-reinvention. I've watched them all age, with curiosity and appreciation for their transformations from girls to women—some more gracefully and honestly than others.

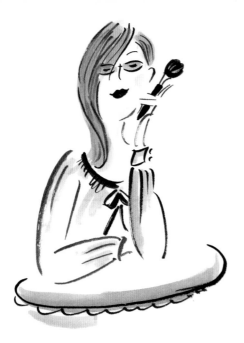

But . . . I've never been someone obsessed—I don't care about their trips to Starbucks or their pet's name, though I do confess to taking special notice of Meryl Streep. I mean, Meryl Streep is ridiculously attractive. Who among us didn't envy her portrayal of a fifty+ divorced woman in the movie *It's Complicated,* as her ex came begging for a second go around, ditching the younger second wife in the process? His slack jaw as Meryl dropped her robe is an image we should tape to our mirrors and embed in our brains, if only to remind ourselves of the last but definitely not least of my exhortations . . .

BEAUTY TRUTH:

Sexy doesn't have an age.

What I *do* think is true about sex appeal and beauty is this: Age is an asset that doesn't erase it; we are more confident now, and we are more appreciative of any physical gifts that we may possess. And after reading this book, we recognize that looking great is the only way to honor those gifts. We know that it is up to us to move beyond inertia to create the persona that matches our vision of how we'd like to present ourselves to ourselves, and to others, every day—it doesn't just happen by accident.

At the beginning of this book I challenged you to look in the mirror, sans makeup—and absorb what you see. Now that we're at the end of our journey together, I am going to ask you to do it again. So, put down this book, look in the mirror, and embrace the lines on your face. And damn it, really do it. Those lines are years of pleasure, tears, madness, and happiness. You have lived it and earned them. Do you remember your first wrinkle? I do. I remember getting my very first crow's foot after crying my broken heart out for days over a boyfriend. Ironically, he told a friend who bumped into him recently that I was the love of his life! Can you imagine? I still have that wrinkle, and he made me work hard for it, and it inhabits me daily, along with the rest of the personal history written on my face. Sometimes I ponder that perhaps I've erased part of my physical legacy with the facelift—but no, I don't think so. There are enough wrinkles left to keep that in place.

Personally, I take real pleasure in using the knowledge of cosmetics I have been privileged to acquire through a fantastic career and a good dose of curiosity. I unapologetically embrace and enjoy the feminine ritual of using cosmetics, and I believe that what my mother called "powder and paint" can do more for my face and my soul than any expensive cream. Makeup has real psychic value. On the days when I've made a real effort and someone who loves me tells me I look beautiful, I want to bottle that feeling.

I totally respect that for some women, cosmetics or fillers or plastic surgery have nothing to do with self-expression, but deeply understand how for others of us, a new tube of lipstick can make our day. You, only better . . . that's the mantra . . . think it each time you lift a tube of lipstick or eye pencil or blush compact from your cosmetic pouch. I thoroughly fess up to the notion that I am a very long drawn out makeover in progress, and suspect that if you have finished reading this book you know of what I speak.

Take it from a woman in the know: Some things do get better with age, and *we* are one of them!

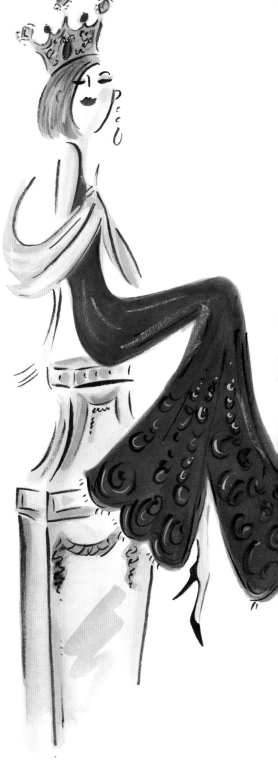

MY THANKS

SINCE THIS BOOK is as much about lessons learned along the winding road of a happy career as it is about the beautiful road ahead for all of us who are fifty and beyond, there are several people I would like to thank for making the path magnificent along the way and seeding it for all the "to comes."

First, not all men are created equal and not all men are "suits." Here are some brilliantly talented men who mentored, supported, and believed in me—I thank you profusely for that: Lindsay Owen-Jones, Alexander Liberman, Irving Penn, Gilles Weil, Ronald Perelman, Bob Nielsen, and Tom Ford, and my deepest gratitude goes to Ralph Lauren and Guy Peyrelongue for providing the happiest eight years of my career.

To some exceptional women who "wore the pants" when it came to creativity, friendship, and encouragement—huge thanks:

To Gloria Appel, my inspiration and cheerleader for so many pages of this book; to my *Mademoiselle* soul mates forever, Nonnie Moore, Sandy Horvitz, Deborah Turbeville, and Edie Locke; to Felicia Milewicz, who supported me on everything; to Midge Richardson, who challenged me on everything; to my *Vogue* best friends, Grace Mirabella, editor extraordinaire, Jade Hobson, and special thanks to my dear friend and beauty colleague Dorothy Schefer Faux, how would this book have been possible without your encouragement?

To my agent at ICM, Kristyn Keene, who stepped up and stepped in where an agent can make magic and you did, and to Andy Barzvi, my former agent, thank you for believing in this project from the minute you saw it and for steering it through its incubation. Thanks also to Andy's able associate, Lindsay Hemphill.

To the thoughtful and wonderful gang at Seal Press, especially my lovely editor, Laura Mazer, and the talented, patient, and kind Merrik Bush-Pirkle, who improved everything I wrote; and to Brooke Warner, who loved and encouraged this project from the outset. I thank you all and ask you in the same sentence—how did you ever put up with my shenanigans?

If a picture is worth a thousand words, then this book should go into the Guinness Book of World Records. Chesley McLaren, your pictures say volumes, make us laugh, and add endless charm to my book. Thank you for your creative brilliance. And thank you to Amanda Davidson for your artful thoughts, organization, and hard work. To the production team at Seal Press—Jane Musser and Domini Dragoone—thank you for your collaborative spirit and creative book design.

To Ali MacGraw, who "tossed the gloss" long before this book was a concept, thank you for that—and to my readers, I say: You should know Ali's beauty is only trumped—no, scratch that, magnified—by her facile mind, her sense of humor, and the joy she takes in life.

I have the pleasure of knowing the best of the best experts and reaping the bounty of their wisdom, knowledge, and love of their expertise—that's why they are so good. Thank you, Dr. David Rosenberg, Dr. Michelle Warren, Dr. Gervaise Gerstner, Louis Licari, and Gad Cohen—I am honored by your presence in this book.

To Susan Trumpbour, Mary Maclean, Faran Krentcil, Claudia Herr, Fiorella Valdesolo, Kristina Stewart Ward, Dana Wood, Dale Burg, Karen Wilder, Holly Siegel, and Betty Beaument—I am so grateful for your valuable research, edits, suggestions, input, and general turns on a dime that you all made to bring shape to this book.

Last, I firmly assert that it does take a village and words cannot express the deep debt of gratitude to my family and friends, without whom I could not breathe. Thank you particularly to my friends Lara Modjeski, Pamela Pilkonis, Daniela Morera, Geoff Donaldson, and Jack Wiswall; and to my talented and brilliant son, Lucius—even though a mother should never brag, one and all, your gift of time, talent, and instinct helped enormously to bring this project into being.

ABOUT ANDREA Q. ROBINSON

A NDREA ROBINSON IS legendary in the fashion and beauty business.

In a career spanning more than forty years, she's revolutionized the way women look and the way they feel about beauty. From her early days as beauty editor of *Vogue*, fashion editor of *Mademoiselle*, and creative director of *Seventeen* magazine, to more recently managing the Ralph Lauren beauty brand and building the Tom Ford beauty business from scratch, Andrea has earned a reputation for always being an innovator. Andrea's personal mission in the beauty business has been to help women look like themselves, only better. This concept has driven her revolutionary beauty industry trends and fostered her passionate interest in cosmetics for her generation.

Andrea modernized the business of cosmetics by inventing the "naked" (or natural) makeup trend and the longwearing lipstick trend when she was president of Ultima II—

both major beauty concepts that continue to engage the interest of women.

Andrea is also a business leader. As president of Ralph Lauren Fragrances, she worked hand-in-hand with Ralph Lauren during an eight-year period of unprecedented growth. She went on to launch the Tom Ford Fragrance and Beauty business for Estée Lauder—in addition to assuming the role of Chief Marketing Officer at Estée Lauder.

Andrea has served on the boards of Cosmetic Executive Women and The Fashion Group International, and has been recognized as an innovative business leader with multiple awards such as Cosmetic Executive Women's Legend and Leaders Award, Women's Wear Daily's Marketing Innovator of the Year Award, and several FIFI awards (the Oscars of the beauty industry) for "Fragrance Star of the Year."

Andrea has two adult children and lives in New York City.

SELECTED TITLES FROM SEAL PRESS

Yogalosophy: 28 Days to the Ultimate Mind-Body Makeover, by Mandy Ingber. $18.00, 978-1-58005-445-4. Celebrity yoga instructor Mandy Ingber offers a realistic, flexible, daily plan that will help readers transform their minds, their bodies, and their lives.

For Keeps: Women Tell the Truth About Their Bodies, Growing Older, and Acceptance, edited by Victoria Zackheim. $15.95, 978-1-58005-204-7. This inspirational collection of personal essays explores the relationship that aging women have with their bodies.

The 3-Day Reset: Restore Your Cravings For Healthy Foods in Three Easy, Empowering Days, by Pooja Mottl. $22.00, 978-1-58005-527-7. These 10 simple resets target and revamp your eating habits in practical, three-day increments.

Rescue Me, He's Wearing a Moose Hat: And 40 Other Dates After 50, by Sherry Halperin. $13.95, 978-1-58005-068-5. The hilarious account of a woman who finds herself back in the dating scene after midlife.

About Face: Women Write about What They See When They Look in the Mirror, edited by Anne Burt and Christina Baker Kline. $15.95, 978-1-58005-246-7. 25 women writers candidly examine their own faces—and each face has a story to tell.

Hot & Heavy: Fierce Fat Girls on Life, Love & Fashion, by Virgie Tovar. $16.00, 978-1-58005-438-6. A fun, fresh anthology that celebrates positive body image, feeling comfortable in one's own skin, and being fabulously fine with being fat.

Find Seal Press Online
www.SealPress.com
www.Facebook.com/SealPress
Twitter: @SealPress